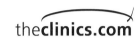

THORACIC SURGERY CLINICS

Current Surgical Management of Pulmonary Metastases

GUEST EDITOR
Robert J. Downey, MD

CONSULTING EDITOR
Mark K. Ferguson, MD

May 2006 • Volume 16 • Number 2

SAUNDERS

An Imprint of Elsevier, Inc.
PHILADELPHIA   LONDON   TORONTO   MONTREAL   SYDNEY   TOKYO

W.B. SAUNDERS COMPANY

A Division of Elsevier Inc.

1600 John F. Kennedy Boulevard, Suite 1800 • Philadelphia, Pennsylvania 19103-2899

http://www.theclinics.com

THORACIC SURGERY CLINICS **Volume 16, Number 2**
May 2006 **ISSN 1547-4127**
Editor: Catherine Bewick **ISBN 1-4160-3560-5**

The ideas and opinions expressed in *Thoracic Surgery Clinics* do not necessarily reflect those of the Publisher. The Publisher does not assume any responsibility for any injury and/or damage to persons or property arising out of or related to any use of the material contained in this periodical. The reader is advised to check the appropriate medical literature and the product information currently provided by the manufacturer of each drug to be administered to verify the dosage, the method and duration of administration, or contraindications. It is the responsibility of the treating physician or other health care professional, relying on independent experience and knowledge of the patient, to determine drug dosages and the best treatment for the patient. Mention of any product in this issue should not be construed as endorsement by the contributors, editors, or the Publisher of the product or manufacturers' claims.

Thoracic Surgery Clinics (ISSN 1547-4127) is published quarterly by the W.B. Saunders, 360 Park Avenue South, New York, NY 10010-1710. Months of publication are February, May, August, and November. Business and editorial offices: 1600 John F. Kennedy Boulevard, Suite 1800, Philadelphia, PA 19103-2899. Accounting and Circulation Offices: 6277 Sea Harbor Drive, Orlando, FL 32887-4800. Periodicals postage paid at New York, NY, and additional mailing offices. Subscription prices are $180.00 per year (US individuals), $270.00 per year (US institutions), $90 per year (US students/individuals), $230.00 per year (Canadian individuals), $335.00 per year (Canadian institutions), $115 per year (Canadian and foreign students/individuals), $230.00 per year (foreign individuals), and $335.00 per year (foreign institutions). Foreign air speed delivery is included in all *Clinics'* subscription prices. All prices are subject to change without notice. POSTMASTER: Send address changes to *Thoracic Surgery Clinics*, Elsevier Periodicals Customer Service, 6277 Sea Harbor Drive, Orlando, FL 32887-4800. **Customer Service: 1-800-654-2452 (US). From outside of the US, call 1-407-345-4000.** E mail: hhspcs@wbsaunders.com.

Reprints. For copies of 100 or more, of articles in this publication, please contact Commercial Rights Department, Elsevier Inc., 360 Park Avenue South, New York, NY 10010-1710. Tel: (212) 633-3813, Fax: (212) 462-1935, e-mail: reprints@elsevier.com

Thoracic Surgery Clinics is covered in *Index Medicus* and *EMBASE/Excerpta Medica*.

Printed in the United States of America.

CONSULTING EDITOR

MARK K. FERGUSON, MD, Professor of Surgery, Section of Cardiac and Thoracic Surgery, The University of Chicago, Chicago, Illinois

GUEST EDITOR

ROBERT J. DOWNEY, MD, Associate Professor of Surgery, Thoracic Service, Department of Surgery, Memorial Sloan-Kettering Cancer Center, New York, New York

CONTRIBUTORS

ITZHAK AVITAL, MD, Hepatobiliary Service, Department of Surgery, Memorial Sloan-Kettering Cancer Center, New York, New York

BENEDICT DALY, MD, Department of Cardiothoracic Surgery, Boston Medical Center, Boston, Massachusetts

RONALD DeMATTEO, MD, Associate Attending, Hepatobiliary Service, Department of Surgery, Memorial Sloan-Kettering Cancer Center, New York, New York

ALBERTO DOMINGUEZ-VENTURA, MD, Resident in Thoracic Surgery, Mayo Clinic College of Medicine, Rochester, Minnesota

ROBERT J. DOWNEY, MD, Associate Professor of Surgery, Thoracic Service, Department of Surgery, Memorial Sloan-Kettering Cancer Center, New York, New York

HIRAN C. FERNANDO, MBBS, FRCS, Department of Cardiothoracic Surgery, Boston Medical Center, Boston, Massachusetts

MARCO GROOTENBOERS, MD, Department of Pulmonary Medicine and Surgery, Antonius Hospital, Nieuwegein, The Netherlands

LEE J. HELMAN, MD, Pediatric Oncology Branch, National Cancer Institute, Bethesda, Maryland

JEROEN M.H. HENDRIKS, MD, PhD, Department of Thoracic and Vascular Surgery, University Hospital Antwerp, Edegem, Belgium

FRANK E. JOHNSON, MD, Department of Surgery, Saint Louis University Health Sciences Center, Saint Louis, Missouri; Surgical Service, Department of Veterans Affairs Medical Center, Saint Louis Missouri

MARK L. KAYTON, MD, Assistant Member, Memorial Sloan-Kettering Cancer Center, New York, New York; Assistant Attending Surgeon, Division of Pediatric Surgery, Department of Surgery, Memorial Hospital for Cancer and Allied Diseases, New York, New York

ARA KETCHEDJIAN, MD, Department of Cardiothoracic Surgery, Boston Medical Center, Boston, Massachusetts

CHAND KHANNA, DVM, PhD, Pediatric Oncology Branch, National Cancer Institute, Bethesda, Maryland

KARTIK KRISHNAN, MD, PhD, Pediatric Oncology Branch, National Cancer Institute, Bethesda, Maryland

JAMES LUKETICH, MD, Heart Lung and Esophageal Institute, University of Pittsburgh Medical Center, Pittsburgh, Pennsylvania

KEITH S. NAUNHEIM, MD, Department of Surgery, Saint Louis University Health Sciences Center, Saint Louis, Missouri; Surgical Service, Department of Veterans Affairs Medical Center, Saint Louis, Missouri

FRANCIS C. NICHOLS III, MD, Assistant Professor of Surgery, Consultant Division of General Thoracic Surgery, Mayo Clinic College of Medicine, Rochester, Minnesota

FRANZ SCHRAMEL, MD, PhD, Department of Pulmonary Medicine and Surgery, Antonius Hospital, Nieuwegein, The Netherlands

WIM J. VAN BOVEN, MD, Department of Pulmonary Medicine and Surgery, Antonius Hospital, Nieuwegein, The Netherlands

BART P. VAN PUTTE, MD, PhD, Department of Pulmonary Medicine and Surgery, Antonius Hospital, Nieuwegein, The Netherlands

PAUL E.Y. VAN SCHIL, MD, PhD, Department of Thoracic and Vascular Surgery, University Hospital Antwerp, Edegem, Belgium

KATHERINE S. VIRGO, PhD, MBA, Department of Surgery, Saint Louis University Health Sciences Center, Saint Louis, Missouri; Surgical Service, Department of Veterans Affairs Medical Center, Saint Louis, Missouri

CONTENTS

determine whether there is a survival advantage associated with pulmonary metastasectomy and how best to integrate metastasectomy with medical therapies, primarily induction, and adjuvant chemotherapy.

This article focuses on the incidence of lymph node involvement at the time of pulmonary metastasectomy, the impact on survival, and potential therapeutic implications. There is current agreement that overall survival can be improved by surgical resection of pulmonary metastases in carefully selected patients. However, the presence of lymph node metastases at the time of pulmonary metastasectomy portends a poor prognosis.

This article evaluates the available evidence for the efficacy of combined liver and lung metastasectomy. In addition, selection criteria identifying patients most likely to benefit from this approach are discussed. Surgery offers the only possibility for prolonged survival and is occasionally curative.

Video-assisted thoracic surgery (VATS) and radiofrequency ablation (RFA) are increasingly being used in the treatment of primary and secondary pulmonary malignancies. Although thoracotomy remains the standard of care for the treatment of the patient with limited metastatic disease to the lung, VATS and RFA may be appropriate in the treatment of selected patients. The number and location of metastases within the lung influence the use of either VATS or RFA. In this article, the authors, based on a review of literature and personal experience, make recommendations for the incorporation of these modalities into the care of patients requiring pulmonary metastasectomy.

This article describes the historical development of pediatric pulmonary metastasectomy but demonstrates that progress has been slow in understanding its proper applications. Because many pediatric metastatic tumors are rare, surgeons have grouped together patients of different histologies for the generation and analysis of case series. By examining tumor types individually, however, it is seen that certain histologies (adrenocortical carcinoma, alveolar soft part sarcoma, osteosarcoma) mandate surgical metastasectomy for patient survival. Other pediatric tumors (Wilms tumor, Ewing's sarcoma) are radiation sensitive, and the application of metastasectomy is controversial. In the case of still other types of tumor (neuroblastoma, differentiated thyroid cancer, rhabdomyosarcoma), metastasectomy is seldom performed except in highly unusual situations. Techniques for minimally invasive biopsy and for muscle-sparing thoracotomy are described for pediatric patients.

Isolated lung perfusion is an experimental surgical technique evaluated for the delivery
of high-dose chemotherapy to improve 5-year survival after pulmonary metastasectomy.
Extensive experimental work in animal models has demonstrated superior pharmacokinetics and efficacy compared with systemic therapy. Phase I clinical trials of isolated
lung perfusion found a maximum tolerated dose**** of TNF-α, doxorubicin, cisplatin,
and melphalan, whereas the combination of isolated lung perfusion with a complete
metastasectomy was feasible. The combination of isolated lung perfusion and regional
lung perfusion techniques needs further investigation.

FORTHCOMING ISSUES

RECENT ISSUES

THORACIC
SURGERY
CLINICS

ELSEVIER
SAUNDERS

Thorac Surg Clin 16 (2006) ix

Preface

Current Surgical Management of Pulmonary Metastases

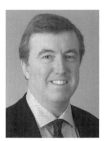

Robert J. Downey, MD
Guest Editor

This issue of the *Thoracic Surgery Clinics* is devoted to the topic of pulmonary metastasectomy—that is, the surgical extirpation from the lung of metastatic disease from extrapulmonary sites. Pulmonary metastasectomy has been widely adopted by thoracic surgeons and is applied to the treatment of a variety of histologies. However, in many ways, the evidence that the patient may benefit from metastasectomy is incomplete and the best means of integrating medical therapies (such as induction or adjuvant chemotherapy) with surgical resection are unknown.

This issue includes articles written by experts in the field who are at the forefront of investigations into the management of patients with pulmonary metastatic disease in an attempt to summarize the state-of-the-art of research into this area of thoracic surgery. I thank the contributing authors for their time and effort in summarizing this area of thoracic surgery.

Robert J. Downey, MD
Thoracic Service
Department of Surgery
Memorial Sloan-Kettering Cancer Center
1275 York Avenue
New York, NY 10021, USA
E-mail address: downeyr@mskcc.org

1547-4127/06/$ – see front matter © 2006 Elsevier Inc. All rights reserved.
doi:10.1016/j.thorsurg.2006.04.001

ELSEVIER
SAUNDERS

Thorac Surg Clin 16 (2006) 115 – 124

THORACIC
SURGERY
CLINICS

The Molecular Biology of Pulmonary Metastasis

Kartik Krishnan, MD, PhD*, Chand Khanna, DVM, PhD, Lee J. Helman, MD

*Pediatric Oncology Branch, National Cancer Institute, National Institutes of Health, Building 10 CRC Room 1-3816,
Bethesda, MD 20892, USA*

Dissemination of cancer cells and the formation of metastatic disease is the single most significant negative prognostic factor in the treatment of cancer. For example, in breast carcinoma, the 5-year overall survival is 96% for localized disease, compared with 21% for patients with metastatic disease. In colorectal carcinoma, the statistics are worse: 91% 5-year overall survival in patients with localized disease compared with less than 10% survival in patients with liver or lung metastases [1]. The goal of routine cancer screening, for example through mammography and colonoscopy, is to identify localized lesions and begin treatment before development of metastasis. Once control of a localized cancer is obtained, adjuvant therapy is aimed at eradication of occult metastatic disease. Despite the advances made in prevention and multi-modal treatment of cancer, however, metastatic disease remains the leading cause of mortality from cancer. Determining which patients and which tumors are at greatest risk for dissemination remain primary goals of the molecular oncologist.

The histological heterogeneity of cancer is reflected in the propensity of particular tumor types to form pulmonary metastases. A large number of tumors (breast carcinoma, osteosarcoma, colon carcinoma, melanoma) metastasize primarily to the lungs. Others (prostate cancer, neuroblastoma), although similar to the former group in their high degree of metastases, only rarely disseminate to the lungs. Still others (nasopharyngeal carcinoma, others) are associated with local invasion but infrequently spread farther than draining lymph nodes. This observation raises two salient questions. First, what causes a localized tumor to become metastatic? And, second, what are the features of the lung that predisposes it as a site of metastatic disease for selected tumor types?

The British surgeon Stephen Paget, in 1889, proposed the first answer to these questions. Paget examined autopsy of records of patients with a variety of primary tumor diagnoses. In contrast to the theory of random dissemination of cancer prevailing at the time, Paget found that metastatic disease fell into a non-random pattern, linking primary cancer type with metastatic target organ. His theory, the "seed and soil" hypothesis, postulates an affinity of factors within tumor cells (the "seed") with factors within the target organs (the "soil"). Although his hypothesis was challenged in the middle part of the 20th century, experiments in 1970s upheld metastasis as a non-random process. As such, identification and manipulation of changes within the primary tumor or factors within target organs may provide a means to abrogate metastatic disease.

More recently, improvements in cellular, molecular and imaging technologies have begun to illuminate the events that occur between growth of a primary tumor to development of clinically or radiographically apparent metastatic disease. Cells from a growing tumor must escape their local environment, travel to the lungs while avoiding clearance from the host, leave the bloodstream, and begin the process of growth. This process requires a complex multi-step sequence of events termed the metastatic cascade. Given the complexity of this progression, events within the metastatic cascade are postulated to be prime targets for intervention in preventing metastatic disease.

---

* Corresponding author.
E-mail address: krishhka@mail.nih.gov (K. Krishnan).

thoracic.theclinics.com

The goal of this review, therefore, is to present the current understanding of differences between the localized and metastatic tumor cell; the biology underlying the lung as the target for metastatic disease; and the molecular and cellular steps of the metastatic cascade.

The metastatic signature

Ideas as to how metastases form from within a mass of primary tumor cells have been postulated since before Paget. Currently, two hypotheses exist in response to this question. The older, and possibly more prevalent, hypothesis holds that cells within a primary tumor inherently have low metastatic potential. Rare cells (as few as 1 in 10^7) undergo somatic mutations during doubling conferring on them a metastatic phenotype through acquisition of such abilities as motility and angiogenesis. These more malignant cells grow within and in concert with the primary tumor but have no intrinsic growth advantage over other less metastatic cells. Once outside the milieu of the primary tumor, however, these rare cells will have acquired the traits that allow them to thrive at metastatic sites.

Evidence of this model of metastasis formation is two-fold. Fidler and colleagues used animal models, wherein poorly metastatic parent cells implanted into mice will form metastases at a low rate. Isolating these metastatic nodules, culturing the cells ex vivo, and re-implantation of these subcloned cells resulted in higher degree of metastasis formation [2]. Furthermore, the long-standing observation that with increased growth of a primary tumor comes increasing likelihood of metastatic disease provides indirect evidence of this somatic mutation model.

The second hypothesis on the formation of metastases holds that the capacity to form metastases is coincident with or very early in the development of the primary tumor. Cells with a metastatic phenotype have a growth advantage over less metastatic cells and predominate within the primary tumor. Ultimately, cells from the primary tumor invade and disseminate to form metastatic disease. This second model is informed by the recent advances in cDNA microarray technology. A cDNA microarray allows for analysis of the expression of thousands of genes at one time. Fluorescently labeled cDNA, isolated from tumor samples, is hybridized to a chip, onto which have been spotted oligonucleotides corresponding to a large number of known genes. Fluorescence intensity corresponds to the presence and amount

(and therefore expression) of cDNA present for each unique gene spot. Comparisons can then be made between primary and metastatic tumors from an individual patient. More importantly, within a specific diagnosis, expression patterns of localized tumors of multiple patients and metastatic tumors of multiple patients could be compared. The resultant difference in gene expression profile from the metastatic versus the localized patients is the so-called metastatic signature.

Recent experiments have validated the existence of a metastatic signature for a number of tumor types. In a study on breast cancer, van't Veer and colleagues used cDNA derived from tumors of a number of patients with and without metastases to develop gene expression profiles [3]. Statistical clustering of gene expression allowed for determination of a 70-gene prognostic set; expression patterns of these 70 genes from primary tumors could be differentiated into bad and good prognosis groups. Further, van de Vijver and colleagues used this 70-gene set to determine if outcome could be predicted based on expression profile. Of the 295 patients analyzed, 180 had poor prognosis signatures. The number of patients with this signature who had developed metastases in the 10-year follow-up period was 50%, compared with less than 15% of patients with the good prognostic signature [4]. Interestingly, this 70-gene signature has been shown to be preserved throughout the metastatic process, because both primary tumors and distant metastases have the same signature [5]. Moreover, Ramaswamy and colleagues provided a broader examination by using metastatic and nonmetastatic samples of a variety of adenocarcinomas [6]. Using a relatively small number of tumors, this group was able to identify a metastatic signature based on expression profiling of primary and unmatched metastatic adenocarcinomas. When applied to a larger set of 279 tumors, this metastatic signature could predict the presence of metastases with a P value of less than 0.03.

Thus, most of the recent evidence has favored the existence of a metastatic signature, usually present at diagnosis, which can identify those tumors at highest risk for development of metastases. In truth, given the complexity of the metastatic process, both models may be correct in different individual patients. Moreover, although the presence of a metastatic signature may be of prognostic significance, and the genes identified may one day be therapeutic targets, no changes in therapy for patients with poor prognostic signatures have yet been implemented.

At the heart of any discussion regarding the genetic origins of cancer or subsets of cancer is the controversy surrounding the existence of the so-called cancer stem cell. A stem cell is a pluripotent cell capable of self-renewal. In cancer, these cells are postulated to be the progenitors from which a malignant mass if formed; they exist within a tumor mass but are often unaffected by conventional cytotoxic therapy [7]. The discovery of cancer stem cells was first made in hematopoietic tumors [8]. More recently, studies on breast cancer have found that a subpopulation of cells within the tumors is capable of tumor initiation, ie, the tumor stem cell [9]. Because these stem cells are capable of new tumor growth, the question of their role in metastasis becomes an important one. Are the malignant cells of a primary tumor and the metastasis, shown to be genetically similar, derived from a population of stem cells located only at the primary site? Or are these stem cells mobile and thus produce malignant disease in distant organs through the same processes as at the primary site? Very limited evidence exists to support either hypothesis, although some work has been performed to suggest that two populations of cancer stem cells exist: a stationary cancer stem cell responsible for precancerous and cancerous lesions at the primary site and a migrating cancer stem cell responsible for metastatic disease [10]. Because the cancer stem cell is not only capable of self-renewal but also of extended quiescence (see "Dormancy"), they may represent the true target of anti-cancer therapy whose eradication is required for any durable cure.

The lung as a metastatic target organ

In 1928, the American pathologist James Ewing began, through his textbook, to challenge the "seed and soil" hypothesis of Paget [11]. Ewing believed that metastasis and their target organs had to do with the anatomy of the vascular system more than any other factor. This view became the prevailing viewpoint of the time and was supported by experimental evidence of Coman and others [12]. The lung, in fact, would represent the ideal metastatic target for a hematogenously disseminated cancer cell. The lung is an end organ with small capillaries, the parenchyma of the lung is, by design, a very short distance from the intravascular space, and the lung is a nutrient-rich environment in terms of blood supply and oxygen tension.

With the elucidation of the selective nature of metastasis in the 1970s, however, the idea that simple mechanical factors are responsible for organ targeting has been replaced with a model requiring a more complicated interplay between metastatic cancer cell and lung parenchyma. The data documented detailing the presence of a metastatic signature raised the question of the existence of a lung-specific (or other organ-specific) metastatic signature. That is, could gene expression profiling identify those cancers that are predisposed to lung metastasis? Initially, the answer was no. Weigelt and colleagues, working with the same breast cancer data sets as those that gave rise to good and poor prognostic profiles, found no indication that gene expression signatures varied depending on the target organ of metastasis [13,14]. More recently, however, Minn and colleagues used breast cancer cell lines injected into mice to select for cells predominantly metastatic to the lungs. They demonstrated that although these cell lines share a gene expression profile with the poor prognostic group, the lung–metastatic lines have a characteristic signature distinct from lines metastatic to bone or adrenal gland [15]. Moreover, the signature of the cells from the primary site of implantation was the same as that of the lung metastases, suggesting the existence of a lung–metastatic signature in these cell lines. Whether a similar signature will be found in human patients, though, remains to be seen.

Whereas genetic factors in the "seed" of metastasis may play a role in targeted dissemination, factors in the "soil" component must also be important. As described, the mechanics of the lung are favorable for metastatic disease. Other organs, for example the kidney, share many similar mechanics and a nutrient-rich environment but are very seldom targets for metastasis. One plausible explanation for this difference is the secretion of attractant molecules by the lungs, molecules which stimulate tumor cells to invade. Chemokines are one such class of molecules. Chemokines are a family of soluble polypeptides responsible for signaling circulating leukocytes to begin the process of transendothelial migration at sites of injury and inflammation. The receptors for various chemokines are present on a large number of tumor types [16]. Among the chemokines produced and secreted by the lung is CXCL12 (also known as SDF-1α). CXCR4, the cognate receptor for CXCL12, is highly expressed on breast cancer cells that show a propensity for lung metastasis. Müller and colleagues demonstrated the potential importance of the CXCL12/CXCR4 interaction in breast cancer metastases [17]. They demonstrated that breast tumor tissue from lung metastases had a higher level of CXCR4 expression than surrounding lung or normal breast tissue. In addition to expression levels, treatment of breast cancer cells with CXCL12 promoted invasion in vitro. Perhaps most importantly, blockage of the CXCL12/CXCR4 interaction with an antibody to CXCR4 significantly reduced the development of pulmonary metastases in immunodeficient mice implanted with breast cancer cells. In addition, the *neu* oncogene (HER2) has long been established as negative prognostic factor and indicator of metastasis in breast cancer. HER2 expression has recently been found to up-regulate the expression of CXCR4 in breast cancer cells [18].

This same chemokine–receptor pair has been demonstrated to play a role in pulmonary metastasis of other tumors. In melanoma, for example, introduction of CXCR4 into B16 melanoma cells induces a 10-fold increase in pulmonary metastases compared with native cells. Moreover, this increase in pulmonary metastases could be blocked by the use of a polypeptide, non-activating ligand mimetic [19]. Blockade of the chemokine–receptor interaction with small molecule inhibitors may yet prove clinically useful to prevent the formation of metastases from a primary tumor. Whether such a blockade would also benefit patients with pre-existing metastases is unknown, but doubtful at best.

The metastatic cascade

Unlike the circulating cancers of the hematopoietic system, dissemination of solid tumors requires multiple steps culminating in the growth of disease at the metastatic site. Various models have been proposed to describe the steps of the metastatic cascade. Here we detail a six-step model. Although the steps of this model differ in their timing and location, the molecules involved in some of the steps overlap. For example, many of the same molecules mediate intravasation into the vasculature as well as extravasation from the vasculature to target tissues. Nonetheless, the progression does occur in a stepwise fashion; differences in the steps may allow for refined molecular targeting efforts to combat metastatic disease.

Intravasation

The process of intravasation, that is, movement of a cancer cell from the extracellular space into the vasculature, requires the cancer cell to traverse the extracellular matrix (ECM) and endothelial basement membrane. Liotta, Kleinermen, and colleagues were the first to document the ability of a cancer cell to degrade the basement membrane [20]. Interestingly, they found that cancer cells collected from the vascular drainage of an implanted xenograft were more effective at degrading matrix components than cells from the primary tumor mass. Likely, this represented the up-regulation of proteases in the disseminated cancer cells compared with the localized ones.

The human genome has more than 500 genes encoding proteases [21]. Of these proteases, many are able to digest proteins of the ECM; the best known and studied with respect to cancer are the members of matrix metalloprotease (MMP) family. MMPs are zinc-binding proteases with the combined ability to degrade any component of the ECM. As such, their activity in normal tissue is tightly regulated. In cancer, however, both the expression and activity of MMPs are up-regulated when compared with corresponding normal tissue [22]. Furthermore, overexpression of MMPs in cancers correlates with reduced survival [23]. Clearly, a primary activity of MMPs is to degrade the components of the extracellular matrix and allow for tumor progression. Recently, though, other activities of the MMPs have been shown to be important in cancer progression. Digestion of matrix components may act indirectly to promote a malignant phenotype through elaboration of pro-metastatic factors from the matrix, eg, cleavage of laminin by MMP-2 results in the generation of a molecule that promotes cell motility in vitro [24]. Furthermore, MMPs act to degrade many pro-inflammatory and immune-stimulating cytokines such as tumor necrosis factor-α (MMP-2) and FasLigand (MMP-9) [25]. Given their ubiquity and importance, the MMPs were one of the earliest targets of anti-metastatic therapy. Preclinical studies with MMP inhibitors demonstrated reduction of metastases in intravenously injected and xenograft mouse models [24]. Unfortunately, the first phase II and III studies with MMP inhibitors, however, have shown no survival advantage [26]. In one phase III trial, in fact, the MMP inhibitor showed a reduced survival compared with standard treatment in pancreatic cancer [27].

In native tissues, MMP function is regulated at multiple levels from transcription through activation by cleavage of the pro-enzyme. Tissue inhibitors of metalloproteases (TIMPs) are small proteins that act to block the activity of MMPs. Overexpression of TIMPs has been shown to inhibit tumor cell invasion [28,29]. Moreover, TIMP gene therapy with adenoviral vectors has shown efficacy in reducing colorectal cancer metastasis in mouse models [30]. Paradoxically, however, high expression of TIMPs in some cancer types is correlated with worse prognosis [31,32]. The control of MMPs, therefore, may yet be an effective target in treating or preventing metastasis, but current approaches are limited by incomplete understanding of the biology of these molecules.

Resistance to anoikis

Non-malignant epithelial cells require interaction with the ECM for survival; loss of this interaction results in the effected cell undergoing apoptotic cell death. Frisch and Francis were the first to document this phenomenon and coined the term *anoikis* (from the Greek for "homelessness") to describe it [33]. In normal tissues, anoikis is a major mechanism for maintaining tissue homeostasis and integrity. Once the basement membrane has been degraded by proteases by a metastatic cancer cell, though, resistance to anoikis becomes a necessity for survival.

In native tissues, anoikis is prevented by two systems: cell–matrix anchorage and cell–-cell interactions [34]. Integrins are the main class of proteins that mediate anchorage of cells to the extracellular matrix. Integrins are transmembrane receptors consisting of α chain and β chain, which form heterodimers on ligation through contact with molecules in the ECM. Formation of these heterodimers triggers an intracellular signal transduction cascade [35]. This signal transduction cascade is initiated through protein phosphorylation and activation of the nonreceptor tyrosine kinase focal adhesion kinase [36]. Ultimately, the cascade results in expression and activation of effectors of growth and survival.

Cell–cell anchorage in normal tissue is mediated by cadherins, a family of calcium-binding glycoproteins. Intracellularly, cadherins form complexes with members of the catenin protein family that link them to the actin cytoskeleton, as well as survival-promoting signal transduction cascades [37]. Loss of either cell–cell or cell–matrix interaction triggers the activation of the caspase proteases, the hallmark of apoptotic cell death.

Metastatic cancer resists anoikis through two mechanisms. The first is through the establishment of cell–cell contacts with other tumor cells (homotypic interactions) or with host cells such as platelets and inflammatory cells (heterotypic interactions). Both homotypic and heterotypic interactions generate intracellular signals preventing the initiation of anoikis.

Additionally, cancer cells may overexpress key proteins that serve to directly inhibit anoikis. For example, the integrin pair $\alpha_v\beta_3$ is frequently overexpressed in malignancy, including prostate cancer and melanoma [38,39]. This overexpression subverts the need for ligand binding and allows signal trans-

duction and expression of survival factors [40]. Moreover, a survey of various tumors of different types and their normal counterparts found that focal adhesion kinase was overexpressed and constitutively activated in 15 of 15 metastatic cancers and 17 of 20 invasive lesions [41]. Furthermore, the adenomatous polyposis coli gene product, APC, has been found to regulate the levels of β-catenin. Mutations in APC allow for unregulated activity of β-catenin, which acts through the Wnt pathway to promote cell growth and survival [42]. Small molecule inhibitors of these components of anoikis resistance are currently being developed [43]. More molecular mediators of anoikis resistance will be discovered and may prove valuable anti-metastasis targets for novel therapies.

Evasion of the immune system

Immunosurveillance, first described in 1909 by Paul Ehrlich, refers to ability of the host immune system to recognize and eradicate tumor cells. Evidence of immunosurveillance comes from the observation that mice lacking an immune system or certain critical components are at increased risk for tumor formation and may also propagate human tumors [44–46].

To survive dissemination, metastatic cancer cells must avoid immunosurveillance at all stages of the metastatic cascade. Cancer cells use a wide variety of mechanisms to effect this evasion. One major mechanism is through the down-regulation of human leukocyte antigen (HLA) class I. HLA class I is the major mediator of immune cell recognition and targeting of cytotoxic T cells and natural killer cells. Not surprisingly, HLA class I down-regulation is associated with invasive and metastatic lesions [47]. Complete loss of HLA class I, however, should result in the activation of natural killer cells because they monitor cells for the presence of HLA molecules [48]. Thus, in addition to, or independent of, the loss of HLA class I, tumor cells may also lose other immunogenic antigens, a phenomenon known as "immunodominance" [49].

Another mechanism by which tumor cells may directly down-regulate the immune system is through the production of immunosuppressive cytokines. Transforming growth factor-β, for example, is a secreted molecule with immunomodulatory activities [50]. Cancer cells and the surrounding stroma often secrete high levels of transforming growth factor-β, with corresponding negative regulatory effects on T cells [51]. Other immunosuppressive molecules are found at high levels in the serum of cancer patients, including the vascular endothelial growth factor and IL-10 [52].

Modification of the immune system remains one of the most studied areas in cancer therapy [53]. These studies have taken the form of tumor specific vaccines and also immunomodulation with cytokines. Neither strategy has proven effective yet. Some new ideas, though, suggest that immunomodulation may play a role. For example, treatment of Ewing sarcoma with a peptide vaccine and adjuvant IL-2 was ineffective in controlling the disease. A reason for this ineffectiveness was recently elucidated as the vaccine induced the production of tolerogenic T regulator cells that may down-regulate the immune response to cancer [54]. Moreover, combine treatment with a pro-inflammatory and anti-inflammatory cytokines (IL-12 and IL-10) were shown to down-regulate growth of primary tumor and metastasis in mouse models of colon and breast cancer [55]. Thus, as we learn more about the interaction of cancer with the immune system, immunomodulation may become an important component of anticancer therapy.

Extravasation

As described, certain features of the lung make it a suitable target for metastatic disease, including chemokine secretion. Moreover, many of the molecules that play a role in intravasation have a role in extravasation, as well. In addition to these, other cell surface receptors play a role in metastatic targeting. Members of the cell adhesion molecule (CAM) family are transmembrane glycoproteins of the immunoglobulin superfamily. CAMs play a role in extravasation by providing linkage of extracellular matrix molecules with other transmembrane receptors [56].

CD44 (also known as H-CAM for homing CAM) is a transmembrane glycoprotein of the CAM superfamily and functions as the receptor for hyaluronic acid in the ECM. In some cancer types, overexpression of CD44 has been shown to correlate with metastatic disease and poor outcome [57,58]. Functional significance of CD44 overexpression was provided by the link between this transmembrane receptor and the membrane–cytoskeleton linker protein ezrin [59]. Ezrin is a member of the ERM (for ezrin-radixin-moesin) family of proteins, initially identified as critical regulators of cell polarity [60]. Ezrin has recently been shown to be critical in the formation of metastasis of multiple tumor type including breast carcinoma, osteosarcoma, and rhabdomyosarcoma [61–63]. Ezrin-mediated signal transduction proceeds through the serine–threonine

kinases AKT and mTOR (mammalian target of rapamycin). Inhibition of ezrin-mediated signaling through the expression of a dominant-negative mutant abrogates experimental metastases in an osteosarcoma model. Moreover, pharmacologic targeting of the AKT/mTOR pathway with rapamycin or its analogs significantly reduced the development of pulmonary metastases in this model [64]. Because rapamycin is currently in clinical trials as an anti-cancer agent, data on its effectiveness at preventing metastasis should soon be available.

Dormancy

Once extravasated and arrested in the target organs, the metastatic cancer cell (or small cluster of cells) may remain as quiescent "micrometastases" for long periods of time. Clinically relevant metastases may present years after successful control of the primary tumor. Thus, these dormant cells are often immune to the effects of standard cytotoxic chemotherapy and radiotherapy.

Multiple mechanisms have been proposed as models of the dormancy phenomenon. The "angiogenic switch" model of dormancy was proposed by Judah Folkman in the 1990s [65,66]. According to this model, small quiescent clusters of tumor cells exist in target organs in an avascular state. This avascularity represents a balance between pro-angiogenic and anti-angiogenic factors that is tilted toward the anti-angiogenic state. Removal of anti-angiogenic factors allows neovascularization and progression of the cells from dormant to actively growing. This model has been re-created in vitro, where dormancy could be induced by anti-angiogenic agents and reversed (leading to growth) by their removal [67].

A second proposed mechanism of tumor dormancy is immune-mediated growth suppression. According to this model, dormant tumor cells reside in an immune-privileged compartment (such as the bone marrow) where they co-exist with a population of T cells [68]. These T cells are CD8$^+$ and maintain equilibrium between the growing cancer and the cytotoxicity of the immune system. At some point through an unclear mechanism, the tumor cells escape this equilibrium and proliferate after first homing to a target organ. Support for this model comes from the observation that transplantation of these CD8$^+$ cells can generate an anti-tumor immune effect in previously unexposed animals [69].

Yet another model of dormancy suggests that cancer cells may leave the cell cycle and become quiescent in response to signals from their extracellular milieu. For example, Aguirre-Ghiso and colleagues demonstrated that dormancy in cells of the head-and-neck carcinoma cell line HEp3 was a response to the ratio of two serine–threonine kinases, ERK and p38^{SAPK}. This ratio was influenced by the activation of α5β1 integrin, focal adhesion kinase, and the epidermal growth factor receptor, demonstrating that the microenvironment surrounding the dormant cells may play a role in controlling quiescence [70].

Given that the process to be observed is lack of cell growth without cell death, models of dormancy are difficult to generate. One recent model takes advantage of advances in in vivo imaging that allow for observation of single cells. Goodison and colleagues found that after implantation of breast cancer cells labeled with green fluorescent protein into the mammary glands of mice, single cells could be detected on the surface of lungs. These cells were present after the resection of the primary tumor and even in the absence of clinically apparent metastases. Furthermore, these single cells could be induced to grow in culture and would form tumors with orthotopic implantation [71]. Whether this model represents true dormancy or an experimentally generated phenomenon, though, remains to be seen.

Proliferation

Proliferation of the metastatic cancer focus requires a blood supply to provide nutrients. In normal tissues, angiogenesis occurs through proliferation of endothelial cells. Endothelial proliferation is a tightly regulated balance between pro-angiogenic factors, eg, vascular endothelial growth factor (VEGF), fibroblast growth factor, and IL-8, and their antagonists, eg, thrombospondin-1, maspin, and angiostatin. Cancer cells achieve neovascularization by shifting this balance toward the pro-angiogenic factors [72]. This shifting balance is a result of genetic and epigenetic factors. For example, expression of oncogenes such as *src*, *ras*, and *TrkB* has been shown to up-regulate VEGF. Also, independent of the presence of oncogenes, the angiogenic balance in a tumor is affected by the cell type of origin and the presence of additional genetic effects such as loss of p53 or p16 [73,74]. Once the "'angiogenic switch" is thrown, however, quiescent micrometastases progress into clinically apparent gross metastases.

Given the importance of angiogenesis in the proliferation of cancer, inhibition of angiogenesis is the subject of intensive investigation. Inhibition of angiogenesis can take the form of direct or indirect inhibitors. Direct inhibitors function by preventing the function of pro-angiogenic molecules. Indirect inhibitors act to block signal transduction pathways upstream of the direct pathways. The most well-known of the direct inhibitors of angiogenesis is bevacizumab (Avastin), the anti-VEGF monoclonal antibody. A randomized trial of patients with metastatic colon cancer comparing chemotherapy plus bevacizumab versus placebo showed that the group receiving bevacizumab had a median progression-free survival of 10 months, compared with 6 months with the placebo group [75,76]. The current class of indirect inhibitors acts to block the epidermal growth factor receptor, which has been shown to increase production of VEGF by tumor cells [77]. Examples of these inhibitors include the small molecules gefitinib (Iressa) and erlotinib (Tarceva), and the anti-epidermal growth factor receptor antibody cetuximab (Erbitux). The early results from trials on these drugs have been modest at best [78]. These trials, however, enrolled patients with advanced disease almost exclusively. Likely, the effect of angiogenesis inhibition will be earlier in the course of cancer to prevent a flipping of the "angiogenic switch."

Summary

Curing cancer requires the treatment of metastatic disease. Whether this is a patient with advanced disease and clinically apparent metastases, or if the patient with localized disease is at risk for development of dissemination, failure to control metastasis will result in a poor outcome. Here, we have presented a molecular guide to our current understanding of the processes underlying metastasis. Experimental clinical trials designed to further the understanding of metastasis are often limited by selection of patients with advanced disease. Therefore, our understanding of the processes involved in the metastatic cascade is limited by the availability of comprehensive experimental model systems. The study of metastasis relies most heavily on xenografts, tumors using human cell lines, or tumor tissue that can grow in mice. These models present a limited recapitulation of the patients. Xenograft models require some degree of immunosuppression on the part of the host, because mice with native immune systems will reject transplanted human tumors, preventing their growth. As a result, mice with immune defects ranging from depleted T cells (nude mice) to absent T, B, and NK cells (SCID-Beige) are used as hosts. As the evasion of the immune system is a key function demonstrated by the metastatic cancer cell, xenograft models, by necessity, subvert this step. Furthermore, recent studies have established that angiogenesis in transplanted tumors is different than in native tumors [79,80], further highlighting the limitations of these models.

With these limitations, studies of metastasis may require development of models of autochthonous tumors, that is, tumors originating in the study animals. A number of cell lines of autochthonous murine tumors have been established that generate metastatic disease after implantation into mice. Moreover, some transgenic animals spontaneously develop metastatic tumors that, although occurring in genetically engineered animals, may represent the most complete model from early development to late effects. Finally, a very promising field of autochthonous tumor studies lies in work with companion animals (pets). Some dogs will have cancer, often with striking similarities to those of their human counterparts. These pets may represent an important study group, because they have autochthonous tumors, occurring spontaneously, in an outbred population [81]. In all of these cases, the tumor, new vasculature, and the immune system are syngeneic with the host.

In addition to the advances in model systems, advances in technology will further our understanding and ability to combat metastatic disease. As demonstrated, genomics is proving to be a powerful tool in identifying those at risk for metastasis. From these genetic signatures, molecular targets may be deduced from the genes altered in patients with poor prognoses. Furthermore, other molecular tools such as proteomic analysis may provide further information [82]. Clearly, therefore, a synthesis of different technologies and complimentary information will be required to target metastases and improve the outcome for patients affected by them.

References

[1] Ries L, Eisner M, Kosary C, et al, editors. SEER Cancer Statistics Review, 1975–2002. Bethesda, (MD): National Cancer Institute; 2005.

[2] Fidler IJ, Kripke ML. Metastasis results from preexisting variant cells within a malignant tumor. Science 1977;197:893–5.

[3] van 't Veer LJ, Dai H, van de Vijver MJ, et al. Gene expression profiling predicts clinical outcome of breast cancer. Nature 2002;415:530–6.

[4] van de Vijver MJ, He YD, van't Veer LJ, et al. A gene-expression signature as a predictor of survival in breast cancer. N Engl J Med 2002;347:1999–2009.

[5] Weigelt B, Hu Z, He X, et al. Molecular portraits and 70-gene prognosis signature are preserved throughout the metastatic process of breast cancer. Cancer Res 2005;65:9155–88.

[6] Ramaswamy S, Ross KN, Lander ES, et al. A molecular signature of metastasis in primary solid tumors. Nat Genet 2003;33:49–54.

[7] Reya T, Morrison SJ, Clarke MF, et al. Stem cells, cancer, and cancer stem cells. Nature 2001;414:105–11.

[8] Lapidot T, Sirard C, Vormoor J, et al. A cell initiating human acute myeloid leukaemia after transplantation into SCID mice. Nature 1994;367:645–8.

[9] Al-Hajj M, Wicha MS, Benito-Hernandez A, et al. Prospective identification of tumorigenic breast cancer cells. Proc Natl Acad Sci USA 2003;100:3983–8.

[10] Brabletz T, Jung A, Spaderna S, et al. Opinion: migrating cancer stem cells - an integrated concept of malignant tumour progression. Nat Rev Cancer 2005;5:744–9.

[11] Ewing J. Neoplastic Diseases: A Textbook on Tumors. 3rd edition. Philadelphia: WB Saunders, Co.; 1928.

[12] Coman DR, de Long R, McCutcheon M. Studies on the mechanisms of metastasis; the distribution of tumors in various organs in relation to the distribution of arterial emboli. Cancer Res 1951;11:648–51.

[13] Weigelt B, Wessels LF, Bosma AJ, et al. No common denominator for breast cancer lymph node metastasis. Br J Cancer 2005;93:924–32.

[14] Weigelt B, Glas AM, Wessels LF, et al. Gene expression profiles of primary breast tumors maintained in distant metastases. Proc Natl Acad Sci USA 2003;100:15901–5.

[15] Minn AJ, Gupta GP, Siegel PM, et al. Genes that mediate breast cancer metastasis to lung. Nature 2005;436:518–24.

[16] Wang JM, Deng X, Gong W, et al. Chemokines and their role in tumor growth and metastasis. J Immunol Methods 1998;220:1–17.

[17] Muller A, Homey B, Soto H, et al. Involvement of chemokine receptors in breast cancer metastasis. Nature 2001;410:50–6.

[18] Li YM, Pan Y, Wei Y, et al. Upregulation of CXCR4 is essential for HER2-mediated tumor metastasis. Cancer Cell 2004;6:459–69.

[19] Murakami T, Maki W, Cardones AR, et al. Expression of CXC chemokine receptor-4 enhances the pulmonary metastatic potential of murine B16 melanoma cells. Cancer Res 2002;62:7328–34.

[20] Liotta LA, Kleinerman J, Catanzaro P, et al. Degradation of basement membrane by murine tumor cells. J Natl Cancer Inst 1977;58:1427–31.

[21] Puente XS, Sanchez LM, Overall CM, et al. Human and mouse proteases: a comparative genomic approach. Nat Rev Genet 2003;4:544–58.

[22] Chambers AF, Matrisian LM. Changing views of the role of matrix metalloproteinases in metastasis. J Natl Cancer Inst 1997;89:1260–70.

[23] Zucker S, Vacirca J. Role of matrix metalloproteinases (MMPs) in colorectal cancer. Cancer Metastasis Rev 2004;23:101–17.

[24] Wagenaar-Miller RA, Gorden L, Matrisian LM. Matrix metalloproteinases in colorectal cancer: is it worth talking about? Cancer Metastasis Rev 2004;23:119–35.

[25] Folgueras AR, Pendas AM, Sanchez LM, et al. Matrix metalloproteinases in cancer: from new functions to improved inhibition strategies. Int J Dev Biol 2004;48: 411–24.

[26] Coussens LM, Fingleton B, Matrisian LM. Matrix metalloproteinase inhibitors and cancer: trials and tribulations. Science 2002;295:2387–92.

[27] Moore MJ, Hamm J, Dancey J, et al. Comparison of gemcitabine versus the matrix metalloproteinase inhibitor BAY 12–9566 in patients with advanced or metastatic adenocarcinoma of the pancreas: a phase III trial of the National Cancer Institute of Canada Clinical Trials Group. J Clin Oncol 2003;21:3296–302.

[28] Albini A, Melchiori A, Santi L, et al. Tumor cell invasion inhibited by TIMP-2. J Natl Cancer Inst 1991;83: 775–9.

[29] Baker AH, George SJ, Zaltsman AB, et al. Inhibition of invasion and induction of apoptotic cell death of cancer cell lines by overexpression of TIMP-3. Br J Cancer 1999;79:1347–55.

[30] Brand K, Baker AH, Perez-Canto A, et al. Treatment of colorectal liver metastases by adenoviral transfer of tissue inhibitor of metalloproteinases-2 into the liver tissue. Cancer Res 2000;60:5723–30.

[31] Aljada IS, Ramnath N, Donohue K, et al. Upregulation of the tissue inhibitor of metalloproteinase-1 protein is associated with progression of human non-small-cell lung cancer. J Clin Oncol 2004;22:3218–29.

[32] Zeng ZS, Cohen AM, Zhang ZF, et al. Elevated tissue inhibitor of metalloproteinase 1 RNA in colorectal cancer stroma correlates with lymph node and distant metastases. Clin Cancer Res 1995;1:899–906.

[33] Frisch SM, Francis H. Disruption of epithelial cell-matrix interactions induces apoptosis. J Cell Biol 1994;124:619–26.

[34] Grossmann J. Molecular mechanisms of "detachment-induced apoptosis–Anoikis". Apoptosis 2002;7:247–60.

[35] Guo W, Giancotti FG. Integrin signalling during tumour progression. Nat Rev Mol Cell Biol 2004;5: 816–26.

[36] Parsons JT, Martin KH, Slack JK, et al. Focal adhesion kinase: a regulator of focal adhesion dynamics and cell movement. Oncogene 2000;19:5606–13.

[37] Fukata M, Kaibuchi K. Rho-family GTPases in cadherin-mediated cell-cell adhesion. Nat Rev Mol Cell Biol 2001;2:887–97.

[38] Seftor RE, Seftor EA, Gehlsen KR, et al. Role of the alpha v beta 3 integrin in human melanoma cell invasion. Proc Natl Acad Sci USA 1992;89:1557–61.

[39] Zheng DQ, Woodard AS, Fornaro M, et al. Prostatic carcinoma cell migration via alpha(v)beta3 integrin is modulated by a focal adhesion kinase pathway. Cancer Res 1999;59:1655–64.

[40] Ruoslahti E, Reed JC. Anchorage dependence, integrins, and apoptosis. Cell 1994;77:477–8.

[41] Weiner TM, Liu ET, Craven RJ, et al. Expression of focal adhesion kinase gene and invasive cancer. Lancet 1993;342:1024–5.

[42] Beavon IR. The E-cadherin-catenin complex in tumour metastasis: structure, function and regulation. Eur J Cancer 2000;36:1607–20.

[43] McLean GW, Carragher NO, Avizienyte E, et al. The role of focal-adhesion kinase in cancer - a new therapeutic opportunity. Nat Rev Cancer 2005;5:505–15.

[44] Pantelouris EM. Absence of thymus in a mouse mutant. Nature 1968;217:370–1.

[45] Kaplan DH, Shankaran V, Dighe AS, et al. Demonstration of an interferon gamma-dependent tumor surveillance system in immunocompetent mice. Proc Natl Acad Sci USA 1998;95:7556–61.

[46] Flanagan SP. 'Nude', a new hairless gene with pleiotropic effects in the mouse. Genet Res 1966;8:295–309.

[47] Garrido F, Ruiz-Cabello F, Cabrera T, et al. Implications for immunosurveillance of altered HLA class I phenotypes in human tumours. Immunol Today 1997; 18:89–95.

[48] Moretta A, Bottino C, Vitale M, et al. Receptors for HLA class-I molecules in human natural killer cells. Annu Rev Immunol 1996;14:619–48.

[49] Schreiber H, Wu TH, Nachman J, et al. Immunodominance and tumor escape. Semin Cancer Biol 2002;12:25–31.

[50] Letterio JJ, Roberts AB. Regulation of immune responses by TGF-beta. Annu Rev Immunol 1998;16: 137–61.

[51] Kirkbride KC, Blobe GC. Inhibiting the TGF-beta signalling pathway as a means of cancer immunotherapy. Expert Opin Biol Ther 2003;3:251–61.

[52] Khong HT, Restifo NP. Natural selection of tumor variants in the generation of "tumor escape" phenotypes. Nat Immunol 2002;3:999–1005.

[53] Mocellin S, Mandruzzato S, Bronte V, et al. Part I: Vaccines for solid tumours. Lancet Oncol 2004;5: 681–9.

[54] Zhang H, Chua KS, Guimond M, et al. Lymphopenia and interleukin-2 therapy alter homeostasis of CD4+CD25+ regulatory T cells. Nat Med 2005;11: 1238–43.

[55] Lopez MV, Adris SK, Bravo AI, et al. IL-12 and IL-10 expression synergize to induce the immune-mediated eradication of established colon and mammary tumors and lung metastasis. J Immunol 2005;175:5885–94.

[56] Okegawa T, Li Y, Pong RC, et al. Cell adhesion proteins as tumor suppressors. J Urol 2002;167:1836–43.

[57] Martin TA, Harrison G, Mansel RE, et al. The role of the CD44/ezrin complex in cancer metastasis. Crit Rev Oncol Hematol 2003;46:165–86.

[58] Wielenga VJ, Heider KH, Offerhaus GJ, et al. Expression of CD44 variant proteins in human colorectal cancer is related to tumor progression. Cancer Res 1993;53:4754–6.

[59] Jothy S. CD44 and its partners in metastasis. Clin Exp Metastasis 2003;20:195–201.

[60] Franck Z, Footer M, Bretscher A. Microinjection of villin into cultured cells induces rapid and long-lasting changes in cell morphology but does not inhibit cytokinesis, cell motility, or membrane ruffling. J Cell Biol 1990;111:2475–85.

[61] Elliott BE, Meens JA, SenGupta SK, et al. The membrane cytoskeletal crosslinker ezrin is required for metastasis of breast carcinoma cells. Breast Cancer Res 2005;7:R365–73.

[62] Khanna C, Wan X, Bose S, et al. The membrane-cytoskeleton linker ezrin is necessary for osteosarcoma metastasis. Nat Med 2004;10:182–6.

[63] Yu Y, Khan J, Khanna C, et al. Expression profiling identifies the cytoskeletal organizer ezrin and the developmental homeoprotein Six-1 as key metastatic regulators. Nat Med 2004;10:175–81.

[64] Wan X, Mendoza A, Khanna C, et al. Rapamycin inhibits ezrin-mediated metastatic behavior in a murine model of osteosarcoma. Cancer Res 2005;65:2406–11.

[65] Holmgren L, O'Reilly MS, Folkman J. Dormancy of micrometastases: balanced proliferation and apoptosis in the presence of angiogenesis suppression. Nat Med 1995;1:149–53.

[66] O'Reilly MS, Holmgren L, Chen C, et al. Angiostatin induces and sustains dormancy of human primary tumors in mice. Nat Med 1996;2:689–92.

[67] Bayko L, Rak J, Man S, et al. The dormant in vivo phenotype of early stage primary human melanoma: termination by overexpression of vascular endothelial growth factor. Angiogenesis 1998;2:203–17.

[68] Schirrmacher V. T-cell immunity in the induction and maintenance of a tumour dormant state. Semin Cancer Biol 2001;11:285–95.

[69] Farrar JD, Katz KH, Windsor J, et al. Cancer dormancy. VII. A regulatory role for CD8 + T cells and IFN-gamma in establishing and maintaining the tumor-dormant state. J Immunol 1999;162:2842–9.

[70] Aguirre-Ghiso JA, Estrada Y, Liu D, et al. ERK (MAPK) activity as a determinant of tumor growth and dormancy; regulation by p38(SAPK). Cancer Res 2003;63:1684–95.

[71] Goodison S, Kawai K, Hihara J, et al. Prolonged dormancy and site-specific growth potential of cancer cells spontaneously disseminated from nonmetastatic breast tumors as revealed by labeling with green fluorescent protein. Clin Cancer Res 2003;9:3808–14.

[72] Kerbel R, Folkman J. Clinical translation of angiogenesis inhibitors. Nat Rev Cancer 2002;2:727–39.

[73] Lopez-Ocejo O, Viloria-Petit A, Bequet-Romero M, et al. Oncogenes and tumor angiogenesis: the HPV-16 E6 oncoprotein activates the vascular endothelial growth factor (VEGF) gene promoter in a p53 independent manner. Oncogene 2000;19:4611–20.

[74] Rak J, Mitsuhashi Y, Sheehan C, et al. Oncogenes and tumor angiogenesis: differential modes of vascular endothelial growth factor up-regulation in ras-transformed epithelial cells and fibroblasts. Cancer Res 2000;60:490–8.

[75] Hurwitz H, Fehrenbacher L, Novotny W, et al. Bevacizumab plus irinotecan, fluorouracil, and leucovorin for metastatic colorectal cancer. N Engl J Med 2004;350:2335–42.

[76] Kabbinavar F, Hurwitz HI, Fehrenbacher L, et al. Phase II, randomized trial comparing bevacizumab plus fluorouracil (FU)/leucovorin (LV) with FU/LV alone in patients with metastatic colorectal cancer. J Clin Oncol 2003;21:60–5.

[77] Goldman CK, Kim J, Wong WL, et al. Epidermal growth factor stimulates vascular endothelial growth factor production by human malignant glioma cells: a model of glioblastoma multiforme pathophysiology. Mol Biol Cell 1993;4:121–33.

[78] El-Rayes BF, LoRusso PM. Targeting the epidermal growth factor receptor. Br J Cancer 2004;91:418–24.

[79] Sikder H, Huso DL, Zhang H, et al. Disruption of Id1 reveals major differences in angiogenesis between transplanted and autochthonous tumors. Cancer Cell 2003;4:291–9.

[80] Alani RM, Silverthorn CF, Orosz K. Tumor angiogenesis in mice and men. Cancer Biol Ther 2004;3: 498–500.

[81] Khanna C, Hunter K. Modeling metastasis in vivo. Carcinogenesis 2005;26:513–23.

[82] Cai Z, Chiu JF, He QY. Application of proteomics in the study of tumor metastasis. Genomics Proteomics Bioinformatics 2004;2:152–66.

ELSEVIER
SAUNDERS

Thorac Surg Clin 16 (2006) 125 – 131

THORACIC
SURGERY
CLINICS

Preoperative Workup and Postoperative Surveillance for Patients Undergoing Pulmonary Metastasectomy

Katherine S. Virgo, PhD, MBA[a,b],*, Keith S. Naunheim, MD[a,b],
Frank E. Johnson, MD[a,b]

[a]Department of Surgery, Saint Louis University Health Sciences Center, 3635 Vista Avenue, P.O. Box 15250,
Saint Louis, MO 63110-0250, USA
[b]Surgical Service, Department of Veterans Affairs Medical Center, 915 North Grand Boulevard, Saint Louis, MO 63106, USA

Resection of pulmonary metastasis continues to be a significant tool in the armamentarium of thoracic surgeons at the present time. At the time of autopsy, 20% to 30% of all patients with metastatic cancer have pulmonary metastases, although most such patients are not candidates for surgery [1,2]. The findings of a large retrospective study of patients with metastatic carcinoma of the colon and rectum treated at Department of Veterans Affairs Medical Center facilities during fiscal years 1988 to 1992 were that only 22% (2659) of the more than 12,000 patients presenting with metastases had pulmonary metastases. [3] Of these patients, only 19% (514/2659) had no previous or other metastatic sites. Only 15% (76/514) underwent pulmonary metastasectomy, resulting in a 5-year survival rate of 36%. Less so in colorectal disease, fewer than 3% of patients presenting with pulmonary metastasis eventually proved to be candidates for surgical excision.

Although this may not be a large public health concern with regard to absolute numbers of patients at risk, it is valuable to determine a "best clinical practice" for the work-up and postopera-

tive surveillance of patients who undergo pulmonary metastasectomy.

This article briefly reviews practice patterns in the evaluation of suspected pulmonary metastases, taking into consideration such issues as local control of the primary tumor, the influence of extrapulmonary metastases, and pulmonary metastatic tumor burden. Further, the article addresses the related topic of surveillance after pulmonary metastasectomy, an area lacking in evidence-based clinical practice guidelines to assist clinicians in the determination of appropriate follow-up.

Workup

The majority of patients are asymptomatic at the time of diagnosis of pulmonary metastases. Pulmonary nodules are generally identified on chest radiography or chest computed tomography (CT) during routine follow-up for the primary cancer. Though pulmonary metastases can arise from a variety of different primaries (ie, colorectal, testicular, melanoma, renal, soft tissue sarcoma, breast), general themes apply to the work-up of all patients with pulmonary nodules detected subsequent to the treatment of a primary malignant neoplasm. Most pulmonary metastases will not be cured by surgical resection, so the first goal is to determine whether the patient will benefit from pulmonary metastasectomy. Thus, preoperative work-up must be designed to determine whether the primary tumor is controlled or control-

The views expressed in this paper are those of the authors and should not be construed as reflecting the official position of the Department of Veterans Affairs or Saint Louis University.

* Corresponding author. Department of Surgery Saint Louis University Health Sciences Center 3635 Vista Ave, P.O. Box 15250 Saint Louis, MO 63110-0250.

E-mail address: virgoks@slu.edu (K.S. Virgo).

1547-4127/06/$ – see front matter. Published by Elsevier Inc.
doi:10.1016/j.thorsurg.2005.11.001

thoracic.theclinics.com

lable. The second issue to be addressed is whether extrapulmonary disease, if present, is controllable. Third, one must assess whether the patient is a fit candidate for major surgery, including whether the patient has sufficient pulmonary reserve to permit complete resection. Finally, alternative treatment strategies such as chemotherapy must be examined to identify the optimal treatment.

Tests commonly used for the work-up of potential pulmonary metastases and the assessment of spread include chest radiography, bronchoscopy, CT of the chest, abdomen, pelvis, and brain, magnetic resonance imaging (MRI), bone scan, and in some cases tumor markers specific to the original primary (serum carcinoembryonic antigen levels, serum alpha fetoprotein, serum hormone assays). Positron emission tomography (PET) with 18-fluoro-2-deoxyglucose (FDG) is a newer modality and is occasionally used but is very expensive, and its cost-effectiveness has been questioned. The work-up of patients suspected of having pulmonary metastases is complicated by the fact that a high percentage of pulmonary metastases are too small (6 mm or less at presentation) to detect reliably using current diagnostic technology. In addition, many lesions identified by imaging tests prove to be benign.

Surveys of current practice patterns in this area are few. The two that were identified focused on pulmonary metastases from melanoma [4] and rectal cancer [unpublished research]. For melanoma, a random sample of the membership of the American Society of Plastic and Reconstructive Surgeons (ASPRS) was selected in 1998 to suggest appropriate testing for an asymptomatic healthy patient who is 1 year status post curative resection of a T2N0M0 melanoma of the forearm (wide local excision with skin grafting and 0/12 lymph nodes involved after ipsilateral axillary dissection). A routine follow-up chest radiograph revealed 40 0.5 to 1.0 cm radiodensities in both lung fields suggestive of metastases. The tests most often suggested in order of frequency of use were complete blood count (CBC) (77%), CT of the chest (75%), serum transaminase level (65%), biopsy of the chest lesions (60%), CT of the abdomen (58%), and CT of the brain (53%).

For rectal cancer, the entire membership of the American Society of Colon and Rectal Surgeons was asked in 2002 to address the following scenario:

> Consider a generally healthy patient who returns 2 years after potentially curative low anterior resection of a T3N0M0 adenocarcinoma of the rectum. No adjuvant therapy was given. On routine follow-up chest radiography he/she now has four 0.5- to 1.0-cm radiodensities in both lung fields suggestive

of metastases. He/she has a serum carcinoembryonic antigen level of 1.4 ng/dL. The patient states he/she feels well overall. His/her physical examination is unremarkable. Which studies would you use in your initial workup?

The tests recommended most often in order of frequency of use were CT of the chest (90%), CT of the abdomen and pelvis (74%), colonoscopy (55%), liver function tests (54%), CBC (54%), serum carcinoembryonic antigen (CEA) levels (52%), and whole-body PET scan (50.7%) [unpublished research].

Distinguishing pulmonary metastases from new primary lung cancer can be difficult. Current criteria for diagnosis of a second primary in the lung are that the tumor must be solitary and histologically distinct from the primary or the tumor must have occurred at least 3 years after diagnosis of the primary [5]. If the patient were treated with wedge resection, as would be appropriate for pulmonary metastases, and was later determined to have had a new primary, wedge resection would clearly have been inappropriate treatment. Genetic markers are needed to confidently distinguish between metastases and primary solitary nodules.

Is the primary tumor controlled or controllable?

Primary site CT is generally recommended. Additional work-up tests to address this question are based on the tumor site such as CEA and colonoscopy or barium enema (colorectal), serum beta human chorionic gonadotropin (germ cell), and serum hormone assays (endocrine). Consultation with the specialist treating the primary tumor is crucial.

Is extrathoracic disease present?

Because patients often have extrathoracic metastases in addition to pulmonary metastases at presentation, and because such patients are rarely candidates for pulmonary metastasectomy, it is important to screen for those extrathoracic metastases most likely to occur based on the initial tumor site. Common tests used for this purpose include abdominal and pelvic CT and brain CT or MRI. Less commonly used tests include bone scan and whole-body CT or PET.

Patients with surgically treated colorectal primaries and subsequent metastases to both the liver and lung are an exception [6–10]. Although the impact of the sequencing of therapy for metastases on survival is still undergoing debate because of small sample sizes in the existing studies, it has generally been found that patients with liver and lung metastases treated sequentially have better outcomes than patients with liver and lung metastases treated synchronously [6,9].

Can the patient tolerate pulmonary resection?

Assessing ability to tolerate pulmonary resection is no different for the patient with pulmonary metastases than it is for the patient with a primary lung tumor. Cardiac stress evaluation and pulmonary function tests are generally used to determine if cardiopulmonary reserve is adequate. Those patients with a history of coronary artery disease, valvular heart disease, or current significant symptoms or risk factors are usually offered cardiac evaluation and echocardiogram. All patients should undergo pulmonary function testing that generally includes forced vital capacity (FVC), forced expiratory volume in 1 second (FEV_1), maximum midexpiratory flow (MMEF), maximum voluntary ventilation (MVV), diffusing lung capacity for carbon monoxide (DLCO) and arterial blood gases (ABGs). A ventilation perfusion lung scan may also be indicated depending on the extent of the proposed resection and the patient's lung function [11].

The ability of pulmonary function testing to detect postoperative complications has been questioned. [12–14] Based on retrospective analyses, Rao and colleagues [12] suggest that exercise oximetry may be a better predictor of postoperative complications than FEV_1. The sensitivity and specificity of exercise oximetry and FEV_1 were 27.2% and 85.5% versus 16.8% and 86.3%, respectively. Further research is needed to determine if these results are generalizable.

Is complete resection possible?

Though chest CT is considered the standard for assessing the extent of intrathoracic spread of the pulmonary metastases, many nodules remain undetected until thoracotomy. Previous studies have shown that helical CT detects approximately 20% more nodules than conventional CT. Margaritora and colleagues [15] compared 166 patients with pulmonary metastases, 78 of whom underwent preoperative high-resolution CT (HRCT) and 88 patients underwent preoperative helical CT (HCT). All patients underwent axillary thoracotomy. Based on the 188 malignant nodules detected at thoracotomy, the sensitivity of HRCT and HCT was 75% and 82.1%,

respectively. Sensitivity decreases substantially with the size of the lesion. For metastases larger than 10 mm, sensitivity was 100% for both groups. For metastases 6 to 10 mm in size, sensitivity was 66% and 68%, respectively. For metastases smaller than 6 mm, sensitivity was 48% and 61.5%, respectively.

In a somewhat smaller study, Parsons and colleagues [16] found 22% more nodules during palpation intraoperatively than were detected by helical CT. The sensitivity of helical CT was 78%. Though the sample size of this study was quite small (34 patients, 41 pulmonary metastasectomies, 88 malignant nodules), the sensitivity estimate is quite similar to that found by Margaritora and colleagues [15].

Though used less frequently because of limited availability and high cost, PET is more accurate than CT in detecting metastatis in mediastinal lymph nodes [17–20] but is unable to detect nodes smaller than 8 mm. Some have suggested that PET be reserved for only those patients with node negative CT scans [21]. The new hybrid PET/CT is believed to be the most comprehensive imaging tool for detecting lung cancer; however, it is still in the development phase [22]. In preliminary testing of numerous tumor sites, PET/CT impacted the management of 14% of the 204 patients studied [23].

It is important that bronchoscopy be performed on all patients to ensure the absence of endobronchially visible lesions. Such lesions are typically found in 2% to 3% of patients and generally lead to a change in the operative approach or the extent of the planned resection, and perhaps even result in cancellation of the procedure entirely if the patient is unable to tolerate a more extensive resection [24].

Such endobronchial lesions have been reported in colon, breast, germ cell, renal cell, and melanomas. The goal is to permit a complete resection while removing the minimal amount of functioning lung in anticipation of recurrence and possible future resections. For unilateral lesions, posterolateral thoracotomy is the standard surgical approach. For bilateral lesions, median sternotomy, bilateral anterolateral thoracotomy (clamshell), and staged, bilateral, posterolateral thoracotomy are the options.

For patients with large proximal tumors or for any patient undergoing resection of metastatic breast cancer, mediastinoscopy should be considered [25]. The presence of involved lymph nodes generally suggests the need to abort the pulmonary resection because complete resection will be difficult to achieve.

Patients who are not candidates for complete resection generally have poor outcomes. Further surgery is only undertaken if there is the possibility of palliation of symptoms to improve quality of life.

Such cases include bronchial obstruction and distal pulmonary suppuration [25].

Examination of Alternative Treatment Strategies

Surgical resection remains the primary treatment for most solid tumors that metastasize to the lung because of the relative insensitivity of such tumors to currently available chemotherapy regimens. Non-seminomatous germ cell tumors (NSGCT) are an exception. For NSGCT, the role of pulmonary metastasectomy has changed from that of primary treatment modality to salvage therapy [26]. Platinum-based chemotherapy regimens are now available that provide curative intent treatment to more than 80% of patients with metastatic NSGCT. Only 5% to 10% of patients with NSGCT still require pulmonary metas-tasectomy [27,28]. Currently, no test reliably predicts the histology of residual pulmonary lesions after initial chemotherapy for metastatic NSGCT [29]. However, one study showed that necrosis at retro-peritoneal lymph node dissection after initial chemo-therapy for metastatic NSGCT was highly predictive (89% probability) of necrosis in the lung, thus sug-gesting that retroperitoneal lymph node dissection and thoracotomy should not be performed at the same session. Knowledge of the retroperitoneal his-tologic status may suggest that thoracotomy is un-necessary, particularly if the primary tumor was negative for teratoma.

Currently, all NSGCT patients should be consid-ered for possible resection, keeping in mind the type of chemotherapy regimen the patient has undergone. Patients with a poorer prognosis may have been treated with bleomycin, which can reduce pulmonary function and cause interstitial pneumonitis, leading to fibrosis in 2% to 3% of NSGCT patients [26] and 2% to 40% of all cancer patients [30]. Risk factors for bleomycin-induced pulmonary toxicity are history of smoking, previous chest radiotherapy, total dose ac-cumulation, and the age of the patient [31].

For osteosarcoma, although adjuvant chemother-apy regimens have substantially reduced death rates [32–35], 30% to 50% of patients undergoing chemo-therapy will still have relapse in the lung [36]. The European Organization for Research and Treatment of Cancer and the International Society of Pediat-ric Oncology conducted the "O_3 trial," the results of which suggested that successful metastasectomy was more frequently possible after previous prophylactic lung irradiation (PLI) than after adjuvant chemo-therapy. Yet unclear is the potential impact of whole-lung radiotherapy on recurrence rates among patients at high risk after metastasectomy.

For cases deemed unresectable and for which systemic chemotherapy is not an option, isolated and regional lung perfusion are currently undergoing evaluation [37]. Isolated lung perfusion selectively delivers effective drug concentrations to one or both lungs while minimizing drug levels in other drug sensitive organs, thus avoiding fatal complications. It has been proposed that the focus of future research using isolated lung perfusion should be on those tumors that spread primarily to the lung such as soft tissue sarcomas, osteogenic sarcomas, melanomas, head and neck cancers, and colorectal cancers. Less invasive methods of treatment, such as regional lung perfusion, are currently being examined [38].

Surveillance

Cancer patient follow-up was originally consid-ered palliative care for symptomatic patients with short life expectancies because cure was extremely rare. With the advent of modern surgical techniques in the nineteenth century, curative-intent treatment of cancer patients became possible. By the twentieth century, further research showed that patients who had undergone curative treatment were vulnerable to cancer recurrence in the same or other sites. Therein, the concept of organ-specific surveillance arose [39]. Detection of recurrence and new primaries became primary goals of surveillance. To demonstrate that surveillance after curative intent treatment is worth-while, however, requires that effective treatment be available for recurrences detected during follow-up. Much of the debate in the cancer patient follow-up literature revolves around this issue. In addition, the optimal surveillance strategy is unknown for most cancers, and little is known about how outcomes vary when a chosen surveillance strategy is altered. Phy-sicians appear to adopt the surveillance regimen specific to their training program. This practice is difficult to justify in the absence of definitive studies comparing patient benefit accruing from follow-up regimens of varying intensities.

Very few published articles address the even nar-rower topic of surveillance after pulmonary metasta-sectomy in any detail [6,25,40–44]. The diagnostic tests generally suggested for follow-up include some combination of chest CT, chest radiography, and pul-monary function tests, in conjunction with tests specific to the primary tumor site or tumor histology. For example, for patients treated with curative intent for colorectal cancer primaries who have subsequently undergone pulmonary metastasectomy, additional tests would include serum CEA level, abdominal CT or ultrasound, and serum carbohydrate antigen 19-9 level [6,25]. There appears to be no consensus among these articles regarding the appropriate frequency of most tests. For 5 years of follow-up, the range for each test was 4 to 12 chest CTs, 8 to 20 chest radiographs, and 0–6 pulmonary function tests (only one author recommended). A search of the English language literature did not reveal any guidelines proposed by medical societies to aid clinicians in developing follow-up strategies after pulmonary metastasectomy.

The primary goal of surveillance after pulmonary metastasectomy is to detect recurrence while salvage therapy is still an option. Another goal is the provision of patient education regarding the negative effects of such modifiable risk factors as cigarette smoking, alcohol consumption, and poor dietary habits. In addition, careful attention must be paid to addressing the psychosocial needs of patients and their families. Finally, detection and management of treatment-related toxicities is necessary.

Only one article to date has examined factors that motivate physicians in the design of surveillance strategies and this study focused solely on surveillance after curative intent treatment of an initial lung primary [45]. In a survey of members of the Society of Thoracic Surgeons (STS), belief that early detection of recurrent cancer can enhance the likelihood of curative treatment of recurrence and can also enhance the likelihood of immediate palliative treatment leading to improved survival were factors most frequently associated with variation in follow-up. STS members reported that maintaining rapport with patients and avoiding malpractice suits were also important factors in the design of surveillance strategies, but these factors were proven in further analysis to have no relationship to self-reported follow-up intensity.

In what manner follow-up after pulmonary metastases should differ from follow-up after a primary lung neoplasm is an interesting question. Further research is needed to address this issue.

Recurrence

After pulmonary metastasectomy, recurrence can occur in the lungs, distant metastatic sites, or at the primary site. When resection of pulmonary metastases was first seriously entertained as a treatment option, recurrence in the lungs was common and multiple resections were frequent. This is still true

today. Lung-conserving resections are now standard, anticipating multiple repeat resections.

A meta-analysis was recently conducted of the experience of 18 major European and American cancer centers over a 50-year period [40]. The resulting International Registry of Lung Metastases (IRLM) contains data on 5290 patients treated with pulmonary metastasectomy. Fifty-three percent of patients experienced recurrence, with a median time to recurrence of 10 months. Patients with sarcomas and melanomas had a higher probability of relapse (64%) than patients with epithelial (46%) or germ cell (26%) tumors. Multiple metastasectomies were not uncommon (20%). Patient with sarcomas were more likely to undergo a second metastasectomy than patients with epithelial tumors, 53% and 28%, respectively. Survival rates after a second metastasectomy were respectable (44% at 5 years and 29% at 10 years). One patient in the study had a total of seven metastasectomies.

High recurrence rates in the lungs after metastasectomy are most likely caused by the presence of micrometastases in the lungs at the time of surgery and are not the result of inadequate resection. Pathologic specimens from surgery proven to have negative margins support this theory. Those patients with recurrence at the primary site likely had occult disease at the locoregional site at thoracotomy.

References

[1] Spencer H, editor. Secondary tumors in the lung. 4th edition. Pathology of the Lung, vol. 2. New York: Pergamon Press; 1985.

[2] Willis RA. The Spread of Tumors in the Human Body. 3rd edition. London: Butterworth and Co; 1973.

[3] Wade TP, Virgo KS, Li MJ, et al. Outcomes after detection of metastatic carcinoma of the colon and rectum in a national hospital system. J Am Coll Surg 1996; 182:353–61.

[4] Margenthaler JA, Johnson DY, Virgo KS, et al. Evaluation of patients with clinically suspected melanoma recurrence: current practice patterns of plastic surgeons. Int J Oncol 2002;21:591–6.

[5] Chung KY, Mukhopadhyay T, Kim J, et al. Discordant p53 gene mutations in primary head and neck cancers and corresponding second primary cancers of the upper aerodigestive tract. Cancer Res 1993;53:1676–83.

[6] Nagakura S, Shirai Y, Yamato Y, et al. Simultaneous detection of colorectal carcinoma liver and lung metastases does not warrant resection. J Am Coll Surg 2001;193:153–60.

[7] Patel NA, Keenan RJ, Medich DS, et al. The presence of colorectal hepatic metastases does not preclude pulmonary metastasectomy. Am Surg 2003;69:1047–53.

[8] Saito Y, Omiya H, Kohno K, et al. Pulmonary metastasectomy for 165 patients with colorectal carcinoma: a prognostic assessment. J Thorac Cardiovasc Surg 2002;124:1007–13.

[9] Headrick JR, Miller DL, Nagorney DM, et al. Surgical treatment of hepatic and pulmonary metastases from colon cancer. Ann Thorac Surg 2001;71:975–80.

[10] van Halteren H, van Geel AN, Hart AAM, et al. Pulmonary resection for metastases of colorectal origin. Chest 1995;107:1526–31.

[11] Lewis CW, Harpole D. Pulmonary metastasectomy for metastatic malignant melanoma. Semin Thorac Cardiovasc Surg 2002;14:45–8.

[12] Rao V, Todd TRJ, Kuus A, et al. Exercise oximetry versus spirometry in the assessment of risk prior to lung resection. Ann Thorac Surg 1995;60:603–9.

[13] Keagy BA, Schorlemmer GR, Murray GF, et al. Correlation of preoperative pulmonary function testing with clinical course in patients after pneumonectomy. Ann Thorac Surg 1983;36:253–7.

[14] Cain HD, Stevens PM, Adainya T. Preoperative pulmonary function and complications after cardiovascular surgery. Chest 1979;76:130–5.

[15] Margaritora S, Porziella V, D'Andrilli A, et al. Pulmonary metastases: can accurate radiological evaluation avoid thoracotomic approach? Eur J Cardiothorac Surg 2002;21:1111–4.

[16] Parsons AM, Detterbeck FC, Parker LA. Accuracy of helical CT in the detection of pulmonary metastases: is intraoperative palpation still necessary? Ann Thorac Surg 2004;78:1910–8.

[17] Pieterman RM, van Putten JWG, Meuzelaar JJ, et al. Preoperative staging of non-small cell lung cancer with positron emission tomography. N Engl J Med 2000;343:254–61.

[18] Cerfolio RJ, Ojha B, Bryant AS, et al. The role of FDG-PET scan in staging patients with non-small cell carcinoma. Ann Thorac Surg 2003;76:861–6.

[19] Reed CE, Harpole DH, Posther KE, et al. Results of the American College of Surgeons Oncology Group Z0050 trial: The utility of positron emission tomography in staging potentially operable non-small cell lung cancer. J Thorac Cardiovasc Surg 2003;126:1943–51.

[20] Gould MK, Kuschner WG, Ware C, et al. Test performance of positron emission tomography and computed tomography for mediastinal staging in patients with non-small cell lung cancer: a meta-analysis. Ann Intern Med 2003;139:879–92.

[21] Dietlein M, Weber K, Gandjour A, et al. Cost-effectiveness of FDG-PET for the management of potentially operable non-small cell lung cancer: priority for a PET-based strategy after nodal-negative CT results. Eur J Nucl Med 2000;27:1598–609.

[22] Groen HJM, Sleijfer DT, de Vries EGE. Positron emission tomography, computerized tomography, and endoscopic ultrasound with needle aspiration for lung cancer. Presented at the 41st Annual Meeting, American Society of Clinical Oncology 2005 Educational Book. Orlando, May 13–17, 2005.

[23] Bar-Shalom R, Yefremov N, Guralnik L, et al. Clinical performance of PET/CT in evaluation of cancer: additional value for diagnostic imaging and patient management. J Nucl Med 2003;44:1200–9.

[24] Downey RJ. Surgical treatment of pulmonary metastases. Surg Oncol Clin North Am 1991;8:341–54.

[25] Todd TR. The surgical treatment of pulmonary metastases: multimodality therapy of chest malignancies– update 1996. Chest 1997;112(Suppl 4):S287–90.

[26] Boffa DJ, Rusch VW. Surgical techniques for non-seminomatous germ cell tumors metastatic to the lung. Chest Surg Clin North Am 2002;12:739–48.

[27] Sonneveld DJ, Hoekstra HJ, Van der Graaf WT, et al. Improved long-term survival of patients with metastatic nonseminomatous testicular germ cell carcinoma in relation to prognostic classification systems during the cisplatin era. Cancer 2001;91:1304–15.

[28] Steyerberg EW, Donohue JP, Gerl A, et al. Residual masses after chemotherapy for metastatic testicular cancer: the clinical implications of the association between retroperitoneal and pulmonary histology. J Urol 1997;158:474–8.

[29] Stenning SP, Parkinson MC, Fisher C, et al. Post-chemotherapy residual masses in germ cell tumor patients: content, clinical features, and prognosis. Cancer 1998;83:1409–19.

[30] Jules-Elysee K, White DA. Bleomycin-induced pulmonary toxicity. Clin Chest Med 1990;11:1–20.

[31] Donat SM. Peri-operative care in patients treated for testicular cancer. Semin Surg Oncol 1999;17:282–8.

[32] Glasser DB, Lane JM, Huvos AG, et al. Survival, prognosis and therapeutic response in osteogenic sarcoma: the Memorial Hospital experience. Cancer 1992;69:698–708.

[33] Raymond AK, Chawla SP, Carrasco CH, et al. Osteosarcoma chemotherapy effect: a prognostic factor. Semin Diagn Pathol 1987;4:212–36.

[34] Tsuchiya H, Tomita K, Mori Y, et al. Marginal excision for osteosarcoma with caffeine assisted chemotherapy. Clin Orthop Related Res 1999;358:27–35.

[35] Tsuchiya H, Kanazawa Y, Abdel-Wanis ME, et al. Effect of timing of pulmonary metastases identification on prognosis of patients with osteosarcoma: the Japanese Musculoskeletal Oncology Group Study. J Clin Oncol 2002;20:3470–7.

[36] Whelan JS, Burcombe RJ, Janinis J, et al. A systematic review of the role of pulmonary irradiation in the management of primary bone tumors. Ann Oncol 2002;13:23–30.

[37] Hendriks JMH, Van Schil PEY. Isolated lung perfusion for the treatment of pulmonary metastases. Surg Oncol 1999;7:59–63.

[38] Furrer M, Lardinois D, Thormann W, et al. Cytostatic lung perfusion by use of an endovascular blood flow occlusion technique. Ann Thorac Surg 1998;65:1523–8.

[39] Johnson FE. Overview. In: Johnson FE, Virgo KS, editors. Cancer patient follow-up. St. Louis (MO): Mosby; 1997. p. 3–10.

[40] Pastorino U. History of the surgical management of pulmonary metastases and development of the International Registry. Semin Thorac Cardiovasc Surg 2002;14:18–28.

[41] Mineo TC, Ambrogi V, Tonini G, et al. Pulmonary metastasectomy: might the type of resection affect survival. J Surg Oncol 2001;76:47–52.

[42] Khan JH, McElhinney DB, Rahman SB, et al. Pulmonary metastases of endocrine origin: the role of surgery. Chest 1998;114:526–34.

[43] Chao C, Goldberg M. Surgical treatment of metastatic pulmonary soft-tissue sarcoma. Oncology 2000;14: 835–41.

[44] Inoue M, Ohta M, Iuchi K, et al. Benefits of surgery for patients with pulmonary metastases from colorectal carcinoma. Ann Thorac Surg 2004;78:238–44.

[45] Virgo KS, Naunheim KS, Coplin MA, et al. Lung cancer patient follow-up: motivation of thoracic surgeons. Chest 1998;114:1519–34.

ELSEVIER
SAUNDERS

Thorac Surg Clin 16 (2006) 133 – 137

THORACIC
SURGERY
CLINICS

Surgery for Colorectal and Sarcomatous Pulmonary Metastases: History, Current Management, and Future Directions

Robert J. Downey, MD

Thoracic Service, Department of Surgery, Memorial Sloan-Kettering Cancer Center, 1275 York Ave, New York, NY 10021, USA

Pulmonary metastasectomy has been performed since 1882 and is now a common procedure at most thoracic surgical centers. An understanding of evolution of the rationale supporting the performance of the procedure is necessary to allow an evaluation of the quality of the data supporting or refuting the procedure. The history of the procedure was extensively reviewed by Martini and McCormack [1] and by Pastorino [2] who have contributed significantly to this field. The reader who wishes to have a thorough understanding of this area of thoracic surgery is encouraged to read these reviews from which the following summary is derived in part.

Before 1898, resection of sarcomas of the chest wall included lung resection if involved by direct extension [3]. The first lung resection for blood-borne metastases (which were discovered at the time of the resection of a chest wall sarcoma) was performed by Weinlechner in 1882 [4]. In 1927, Divis [5] was reported as having performed the first resection of pulmonary metastases as a planned, separate procedure. The first report in the English literature of a planned metastasectomy was by Torek in 1930 [6], but this operation was preceded by one performed by Edwards [7] in 1927 but reported in 1934.

The first case series was published in 1947 and consisted of 24 patients; 12 of these patients were free of disease at the time of the report [8]. This series also contained the first report of the resection of metachronous metastases, with the patient remaining free

of disease 14 years after her second metastasectomy. In this and other series following shortly thereafter, most of the procedures performed were anatomic resections such as lobectomy or pneumonectomy. Alexander and Haight [8] also set criteria for resection: (1) the primary site of disease needed to be controlled or controllable, (2) no extrapulmonary metastases should be present, and (3) the patient had to be medically fit to tolerate the resection.

Since then, there have been approximately 500 publications that address the results achieved by the resection of a variety of primary tumor types. Only a few of these reports, however, contain prospectively collected data, and none of the prospective studies include control groups or randomization comparing surgery to best medical therapy. All retrospective data is susceptible to deficiencies such as selection bias. In addition, studies of pulmonary metastasectomy commonly combine patients who undergo varying treatment regimens, differ in induction and adjuvant chemotherapies, and often do not distinguish between histologies (such as liposarcoma and chondrosarcoma, commonly combined as "sarcomas") that may differ in aggressiveness and response to medical therapies.

The strongest evidence supporting the efficacy of metastasectomy dates from the 1970s [9,10]. A review of 145 patients who had extremity resection for osteogenic sarcoma at Memorial Sloan-Kettering Cancer Center revealed that 83% developed pulmonary metastases within the first 2 years, and the survival rates of patients who developed recurrences were 12% at 2 years and 0% at 5 years. Dr. Marcove

E-mail address: downeyr@mskcc.org

1547-4127/06/$ – see front matter © 2006 Elsevier Inc. All rights reserved.
doi:10.1016/j.thorsurg.2006.03.001

suggested to Dr. Martini to consider resection. Subsequently, 22 patients underwent pulmonary metastasectomy with removal of all palpable disease and experienced a 5-year survival rate of 32% and a 20-year survival rate of 18%.

In 1983, the Institute Nazionale Tumori of Milan, Italy, initiated a prospective study evaluating the efficacy of bilateral lung exploration and resection through a median sternotomy [11,12]. When compared with historical controls, the overall survival rate of all patients receiving treatment for osteosarcoma (including resection for some) improved from 35% to 58%, and the overall 5-year survival rate after detection of pulmonary metastases improved from 0% to 28%. For the subgroup of patients who had pulmonary metastases, selective use of resection improved the survival rate at 5 years to 47%.

In 1990, the International Registry of Pulmonary Metastases was formed [13]. Eighteen centers participated, contributing data on 5290 patients who had undergone metastasectomy. The data collected were retrospective and prospective. Analysis of the data allowed the creation of a prognostic model containing four prognostic groups:

Group 1: resectable, disease-free interval
> 36 months, single metastasis
Group 2: resectable, disease-free interval
> 36 months or single metastasis
Group 3: resectable, disease-free interval
< 36 months and two or more metastases
Group 4: unresectable

The median survival was 61 months for group 1, 34 months for group 2, 24 months for group 3, and 14 months for group 4. Although the prognosis of patients who had different histologies (such as osteosarcoma, soft tissues sarcoma, colon cancer, breast cancer, and melanoma) differed, this prognostic model was significant in each histology. Data were collected on patients who underwent repeated lung metastasectomy, with 5-year survival rates of 44% and 10-year survival rates of 29% being achieved. Significant positive prognostic variables for survival after second metastasectomy were completeness of resection, disease-free survival greater than 12 months, and a solitary metastasis.

Based on these data, the author and colleagues perform pulmonary resection for metastatic disease for a wide variety of histologies and reviewed this experience to document a probable survival advantage associated with the procedure for such diseases as metastatic colorectal cancer [14], sarcoma [15], testicular germ cell tumors [16], thyroid carcinoma [17], other head and neck malignancies [18], and renal cell carcinoma [19]. The author and colleagues' data suggest that resection of recurrent pulmonary metastases is warranted [20] (although this has been shown only for a few histologies) and is commonly performed.

Surgical issues

Several surgical approaches can be taken to effect resection, including video-assisted thoracic surgical procedures [21,22], posterolateral thoracotomy, median sternotomy, bilateral anterior thoracotomy, or "clamshell" thoracotomy (bilateral anterior thoracotomy with transverse sternotomy), and these have been recently reviewed in detail [23]. It is not clear which operation should be performed for the patient who has radiologically resectable disease, and reasonable, experienced surgeons have differing approaches. The author's current approach to the patient who has evidence of unilateral disease only is to perform a unilateral thoracotomy. If bilateral disease is likely, then sequential posterolateral thoracotomies, a clam-shell thoracotomy, or simultaneous anterior thoracotomies are performed. The author rarely considers thoracoscopic resection of all radiographic disease appropriate because manual palpation of the lung finds additional sites of disease in 30% of patients [14]. The use of helical CT scans has not significantly lowered this rate of finding unsuspected disease [24]. This approach, however, can be criticized: If it is important to detect and resect all disease, then why not explore the contralateral side at the same operation because it has been shown that contralateral exploration finds disease not evident on radiographs 38% of patients [25]? If we are willing to leave contralateral disease until it becomes evident radiographically, then why is it deleterious to leave disease after video-assisted thoracic surgery in one third of patients on the ipsilateral side? It must be conceded that logically, if the highest goal is complete resection of all possible sites of disease, then bilateral exploration is warranted. If the highest goal is to limit surgical trauma, then for patients who have unilateral radiographic disease, video-assisted thoracic surgery resection of all evident radiographic disease is reasonable. It is unfortunate that the CALGB trial 39804, a randomized prospective comparison of thoracoscopy and thoracotomy that would have allowed an assessment of the relative risks and benefits of these two approaches, closed due to failure to accrue patients.

Many surgeons do not routinely performed hilar and mediastinal nodal sampling or resection. The recent report by Pfannschmidt and colleagues [26] suggested that approximately 25% (80/245 patients will be found to have nodal metastases if complete nodal dissection is routinely performed. The survival of patients who did not have nodal metastases was 64 months, 33 months for patients who had N1 disease, and 21 months for patients who had N2 disease. The investigators did not provide an analysis of whether nodal involvement was an independent prognostic factor from disease-free interval and the number of metastases, as described earlier. It is likely, however, that because delineation of nodal disease may help guide postoperative decision making (including the administration of adjuvant therapy and the likely benefit of further surgery), routine nodal sampling or dissection should be considered.

Although anatomic resections such as a lobectomy were commonly performed in the 1940s to 1960s, it is now commonly agreed that a limited resection such as a wedge resection is adequate for pulmonary metastasectomy; however, the optimal minimal margin for wedge resections to minimize the likelihood of local recurrence has not been defined. If an anatomic resection such as a segmentectomy, lobectomy, or even a pneumonectomy [27] is required to encompass all disease, then it is reasonable to perform these more extensive resections in selected patients.

Future directions

There are considerable opportunities for research in the area of pulmonary metastatasectomy. First, there are issues that could be addressed in any institution performing metastasectomies. For example, elevation of preoperative carcinoembryonic antigen to above 200 ng/mL has been shown to be a negative prognostic factor for survival after liver resection for metastatic colorectal carcinoma [28], but whether carcinoembryonic antigen levels obtained preoperatively define prognosis for patients with colorectal pulmonary metastases has not been investigated. Similarly, although there are now better data documenting the frequency of finding hilar and mediastinal nodal metastases in patients who have pulmonary parenchymal metastases [26], there has been very little work investigating the prognostic implications of involved nodes. Second, there are other issues that can be addressed only by dedicated research facilities, such as the use of isolated lung perfusion in an attempt to treat micrometastases, as described by Hendriks et al elsewhere in this issue.

The two largest issues, however, are first defining whether there is a survival advantage associated with pulmonary metastasectomy and, second, how best to integrate metastasectomy with medical therapies, primarily induction, and adjuvant chemotherapy.

Regarding the question of benefit associated with metastasectomy, as previously discussed, given the limited evidence that is available, it is possible that there is no benefit associated with metastasectomy and that patients who have resectable pulmonary metastatic disease are a subset with favorable prognoses such that they may have enjoyed prolonged survival without surgery. The most coherent articulation of this viewpoint is by Aberg [29]. Definitive proof that pulmonary metastasectomy improves survival for any histology would probably require a phase III trial. The two histologies most commonly resected are colon carcinoma and sarcoma. It is likely that such a trial using patients who have sarcoma is not feasible; even if it could be completed, it would generate information of limited quality and generalizability for the following four reasons. First, the belief of treating physicians that the retrospective data supporting metastasectomy are strong enough makes physicians reluctant to randomize patients to an arm without surgery. Second, such a trial would require approximately 250 to 300 patients in each arm. If such a trial were to be initiated for sarcoma, the limited number of patients who have resectable pulmonary metastases (approximately 500/y in the United States) would make reaching accrual goals difficult. The most recent attempt to conduct such a trial was the European Organization for Research and Treatment of Cancer (EORTC) Protocol 62,933 that randomized patients who had metastatic sarcoma to metastasectomy alone or to induction chemotherapy followed by metastasectomy. This trial opened in 1996 but closed due to poor accrual. Third, the varied sarcomatous histologies (ie, liposarcoma, malignant fibrous histiocytoma, angiosarcoma, and so forth), which are of different behavior, would have to be clumped together because of the limited number of patients available. This grouping of histologies could affect the validity of the results. Finally, even if it were to be shown that lung resection for sarcomatous metastases definitely improved the likelihood of survival, the number of patients afforded benefit is likely to be small. Data from the prospectively maintained Memorial Sloan-Kettering Cancer Center Sarcoma Database show that of 3149 patients seen over 15 years, 719 (23%) presented with or developed lung metastases. Of these, 248 (8% of all patients; 34% of patients who had metastases) underwent complete resection. Of the 248 patients, 60% suffered pulmonary re-recurrence, and half of these underwent a second resection; of these, half again will undergo further resections for re-recurrent disease. Overall, therefore, from the date of diagnosis of first pulmonary metastases, 35% of patients who have pulmonary metastases able to undergo a complete resection will enjoy a 5-year disease-specific survival. It is not clear that results achieved by metastasectomy for sarcoma could be generalized to other histologies.

Therefore, the author believes that pulmonary metastasectomy trials should focus on patients who have the more common problem of colorectal metastases. Given that physicians and patients may be reluctant to participate in a trial in which a patient may be randomized to an arm that does not involve surgery, a randomized trial to test whether there is any benefit at all to metastasectomy could focus first on poor-risk patients (ie, those who have short disease-free intervals and more than one metastasis). If no benefit to surgery is found in this group of patients, then these data could be used to support a trial that includes patients who have better-prognosis disease.

Trials attempting to understand how to best combine medical and surgical therapies in patients who have pulmonary metastatic colorectal cancer are also urgently needed. Data supporting combined modality therapy are available from the more extensive experience with colorectal cancer metastatic to the liver. A collective multi-institutional series established that hepatic resection for colorectal carcinoma provided a 5-year survival rate of 33% [30]. Other studies have demonstrated a 10-year survival rate of 22% and even 20-year survivors [28], whereas historical controls demonstrate few survivors at 5 years and none at 10 years. Recently, oxaliplatin-based regimens have been shown to improve 3-year disease-free survival over 5-fluorouracil/leucovorin in patients who have stage II and III colon cancer [31] and have found a role in the adjuvant therapy after resection of colorectal metastases [32–34]. Extending this work further, there is an evolving role for induction therapy for unresectable colorectal metastases to the liver, with the goal of rendering them resectable [35].

This chemotherapy is also effective against pulmonary metastatic disease [36]; however, it is unclear how to combine modalities. Patients have had induction chemotherapy lead to pathologic responses, and other patients who had complete radiographic responses had rapid recurrences after completion of chemotherapy.

Therefore, a trial could be constructed in which patients who have colorectal metastases (resectable or unresectable) could be treated with induction therapy and then surgery if possible. End points would be radiographic and pathologic response, rate of complete resection, and disease-free and overall survival.

References

[1] Martini N, McCormack PM. Evolution of the surgical management of pulmonary metastases. Chest Surg Clin N Am 1998;8(1):13–27.

[2] Pastorino U. History of the surgical management of pulmonary metastases and development of the International Registry. Semin Thorac Cardiovasc Surg 2002; 14:18–28.

[3] Gerulanos M. Eine Studie uber den operativen Pneumothorax im Anschluss an einem Fall von Lungenresection wegen Brustwandsarcom. Deutsche Ztschr Chir 1989;49:497–536.

[4] Weinlechner JW. Zur Kasuistik der Tumoren an der Brustwand und dern Behandlung (Resektion der Rippen, Eroffnung der Brusthohle, partielle Entfernung der Lunge). Wien Med Wochenschr 1882;32:589–91, 624–8.

[5] Divis G. Ein Beitrag Zur Operativen Behandlung der Lungeschwulste. Acta Chir Scand 1927;62:329–41.

[6] Torek F. Removal of metastatic carcinoma of the lung and mediastinum. Arch Surg 1930;21:1416–24.

[7] Edwards AT. Malignant disease of the lung. J Thorac Surg 1934;4:107–24.

[8] Alexander J, Haight C. Pulmonary resection for solitary metastatic sarcomas and carcinomas. Surg Gynecol Obstet 1947;85:129–46.

[9] Marcove RC, Mike V, Hajek JV, et al. Osteogenic sarcoma under the age of 21: a review of 145 operative cases. J Bone Joint Surg Am 1970;52:411–21.

[10] Martini N, Mike V, Hajek JV, et al. Multiple pulmonary resections in the treatment of osteogenic sarcoma. Ann Thorac Surg 1971;12:271–80.

[11] Pastorino U, Valente M, Gasparini M, et al. Median sternotomy and multiple lung resections for metastatic sarcomas. Eur J Cardiothorac Surg 1990;4:477–81.

[12] Pastorino U, Gasparini M, Tavecchio L, et al. The contribution of salvage surgery to the management of childhood osteosarcoma. J Clin Oncol 1991;9:1357–62.

[13] Pastorino U, Buyse M, Friedel G, et al. Long-term results of lung metastasectomy: prognostic analyses based on 5206 cases. J Thorac Cardiovasc Surg 1997; 113:37–49.

[14] McCormack PM, Burt ME, Bains MS, et al. Lung resection for colorectal metastases: 10-year results. Arch Surg 1992;127:1403–6.

[15] Billingsley KG, Burt ME, Jara E, et al. Pulmonary metastasectomy from soft tissue sarcoma: analysis of

pattern of disease and postmetastasis survival. Ann Surg 1999;229(5):602–12.

[16] Liu D, Abolhoda A, Burt ME, et al. Pulmonary metastasectomy for testicular germ cell tumors: a 28-year experience. Ann Thorac Surg 1998;66:1709–14.

[17] Stojadinovic AS, Shoup M, Ghossein RA, et al. The role of operations for distantly metastatic well-differentiated thyroid carcinoma. Surgery 2002;131: 636–43.

[18] Liu D, Labow DM, Dang N, et al. Pulmonary metastasectomy for head and neck cancers. Ann Surg Oncol 1999;6(6):572–8.

[19] Russo P. Surgical intervention in patients with metastatic renal cancer: current status of metastasectomy and cytoreductive nephrectomy. Nat Clin Pract Urol 2004;1(1):26–31.

[20] Weiser MR, Downey RJ, Leung DHY, et al. Repeat resection of pulmonary metastases in patients with soft-tissue sarcoma. J Am Coll Surg 2000;191:184–91.

[21] Mineo TC, Pompeo E, Ambrogi V, et al. Video-assisted approach for transxiphoid bilateral lung metastasectomy. Ann Thor Surg 1999;67:1808–10.

[22] Landreneau RJ, De Giacomo T, Mack MJ, et al. Therapeutic video-assisted thoracoscopic surgical resection of colorectal pulmonary metastases. Eur J Cardiothorac Surg 2000;18:671–7.

[23] Rusch VW. Surgical techniques for pulmonary metastasectomy. Semin Thorac Cardiovasc Surg 2002;14:4–9.

[24] Parson AM, Detterbeck FC, Parker LA. Accuracy of helical CT in the detection of pulmonary metastases: is intraoperative palpation still necessary? Ann Thorac Surg 2004;78:1910–8.

[25] Roth JA, Pass HI, Wesley MN, et al. Comparison of median sternotomy and thoracotomy for resection of pulmonary metastases in patients with adult soft-tissue sarcomas. Ann Thorac Surg 1986;42:134–8.

[26] Pfannschmidt J, Klode J, Muley T, et al. Nodal involvement at the time of pulmonary metastasectomy: experiences in 245 patients. Ann Thorac Surg 2006;81: 448–54.

[27] Koong HN, Pastorino U, Ginsbert RJ, for the International Registry of Lung Metastases. Is there a role for pneumonectomy in pulmonary metastases? Ann Thorac Surg 1999;68:2039–43.

[28] Fong Y, Fortner J, Sun RL, et al. Clinical score for predicting recurrence after hepatic resection for metastatic colorectal cancer: analysis of 1001 consecutive cases. Ann Surg 1999;230:309–18.

[29] Aberg T. Selection mechanisms as major determination of survival after pulmonary metastasectomy. Ann Thorac Surg 1997;63:777–84.

[30] Hughes KS, Simon R, Songhorabodi S, et al. Resection of the liver for colorectal carcinoma metastases: a multi-institutional study of patterns of recurrence. Surgery 1986;100:278–84.

[31] Andre T, Boni C, Mounedji-Boudiaf L, et al. Oxaliplatin, fluorouracil, and leucovorin as adjuvant treatment for colon cancer. N Engl J Med 2004;350: 2343–51.

[32] Kememny MM, Adak S, Gray B, et al. Combined-modality treatment for respectable metastatic colorectal carcinoma to the liver: surgical resection of hepatic metastases in combination with continuous infusion of chemotherapy—an intergroup study. J Clin Oncol 2002;20:1499–505.

[33] Kemeny N, Huang Y, Cohen AM, et al. Hepatic arterial infusion of chemotherapy after resection of hepatic metastases from colorectal cancer. N Engl J Med 1999;341:2039–48.

[34] Kemeny NE, Gonen M. Hepatic arterial infusion after liver resection. N Engl J Med 2005;352:734–5.

[35] Pozzo C, Basso M, Cassano A, et al. Neoadjuvant treatment of unresectable liver disease with irinotecan and 5-fluorouracil plus folonic acid in colorectal cancer patients. Ann Oncol 2004;15:933–9.

[36] Schrag D, Weiser M, Schattner M, et al. An increasingly common challenge: management of the complete responder with multi-focal metastatic colorectal cancer. J Clin Oncol 2005;23:1799–802.

ELSEVIER
SAUNDERS

Thorac Surg Clin 16 (2006) 139–143

THORACIC
SURGERY
CLINICS

Lymphadenectomy in Metastasectomy

Alberto Dominguez-Ventura, MD, Francis C. Nichols III, MD*

Mayo Clinic College of Medicine, 200 First Street SW, Rochester, MN 55905, USA

The inability to prevent and eliminate metastatic disease remains the principle reason for cancer death. The lung remains a frequent site of metastatic disease, and the presence of pulmonary metastases often portends uncontrollable tumor spread and subsequent death. Since the first pulmonary metastasectomy (PM) was reported in 1882 [1], hundreds of articles focusing on PM have been published. It is now generally agreed that overall survival can be improved by surgical resection of pulmonary metastases in carefully selected patients [2–4].

Nevertheless, survival after resection of pulmonary metastases remains far from satisfactory. Much has been focused on prognostic indicators for patients undergoing PM. Among these indicators are the cell type of the primary tumor, time interval between primary tumor resection and the identification of pulmonary metastases, number of pulmonary metastases, and the ability to completely resect all metastatic disease. Until recently, very little attention has been paid to the influence of lymph node metastases on patient outcomes after PM. This article focuses on the incidence of lymph node involvement at the time of PM, its impact on survival, and the potential therapeutic implications of this finding.

Incidence

Despite mediastinal lymph node dissection or sampling being a widely accepted standard in pulmonary

resection for primary lung cancer [5], its role during PM has not been well-defined. One of the primary reasons for this is the infrequency with which mediastinal lymphadenectomy or sampling was performed in many PM series [6]. It is often noted that the International Registry of Lung Metastases found only a 5% incidence of lymph node metastases in 5206 patients undergo PM [2]. Most importantly, it must be recognized that lymph nodes were resected or sampled in only 4.6% of these patients [2]. Putnam has suggested that mediastinal lymph node metastases rarely occur from pulmonary metastases [4,7]; however, his personal series deal almost exclusively with metastatic sarcoma. Similarly, Pass and colleagues have stated that only rarely are metastases found in regional lymph nodes, and thus formal lymph node dissection is rarely indicated [8]. Martini and McCormick concluded that pulmonary carcinoma metastases are likely to metastasize to regional lymph nodes, especially melanomas. However, they failed to discuss mediastinal lymph node dissection as part of PM [3].

There appears to be consensus that sarcomas metastatic to the lung rarely spread to mediastinal lymph nodes [3,7]. Thus, we focus the remainder of this article on pulmonary metastases of carcinomatous histopathology.

Abrams and colleagues in a series involving 1000 consecutive autopsies on patients with malignant neoplasms found a 33% incidence of mediastinal lymph node metastases in patients with non-pulmonary carcinoma [9]. When analyzed by primary tumor, the authors found an incidence of mediastinal lymph node metastases of 66% in breast cancer, 30% in stomach, 15% in colon, 20% in rectal, 30% in ovarian, and 47% in kidney cancer [9]. What is not clear from

* Corresponding author.
E-mail address: nichols.francis@mayo.edu
(F.C. Nichols III).

Abrams series is how many patients had pulmonary metastases in addition to the mediastinal lymph node involvement.

In one of the first reports of lymph node metastases identified during PM, Thomford and colleagues reviewed our institutional experience with pulmonary metastases in 1965 [10]. They reported on 221 pulmonary resections in 205 patients over a 21-year period. Twenty patients (9.8%) had metastatically involved lobar or hilar lymph nodes. Overall 5-year survival was 30.3%; however, patients with metastatically involved lymph nodes had only an 8% 5-year survival [10]. Finally, Cahan and colleagues presented their results in 31 patients having PM for metastatic colon cancer [11]. Whereas these authors stressed that no extra effort was made to remove lymph nodes, in 20 patients regional lymphatics were available for pathologic review and in 50% of these patients metastases were found.

The incidence of lymph node metastases in these early series is not surprising if one considers that most pulmonary metastases during those time periods were discovered by ordinary chest x-ray and many patients were symptomatic at presentation.

Table 1 shows the rate of mediastinal lymph node dissection as well as the reported incidence of metastatic lymph node involvement in several recent PM series. From these series it is apparent that evaluation of lymph nodes at the time of PM is not uniformly undertaken. In our most recent series addressing PM, Ercan and colleagues found complete mediastinal lymphadenectomy was performed in only 107 of 883 patients (12.1%) having PM [12]. The decision to perform lymphadenectomy was not based on the appearance of lymph nodes at the time of PM, but rather was based on the individual beliefs of the surgeons with regards to the incidence of lymph node metastases at PM.

Attention should be focused on the PM series in which mediastinal lymphadenectomy or sampling was routinely performed [14,16–18] (Table 1). The incidence of metastatic lymph node involvement ranged from 14.3% to 29.8%. All far in excess of the 5% incidence of metastatically involved lymph nodes reported in the International Registry of Lymph Node Metastases [2].

Prognostic significance

Recent articles have investigated the prognostic significance of metastatic lymph node found during PM. Table 2 displays the results of several series published within the past 10 years. Shown is a survival comparison between patients with positive and negative lymph nodes. At the time of PM, if lymph nodes are not metastatically involved, 5-year survival ranges from 24.7% to 50%. This is in contradistinction with metastatically involved lymph nodes in which the 5-year survival ranges from 0% to 24%. In three of these series, after multivariate analysis lymph node status remained a significant independent prognostic factor [17,19,21].

In our series, overall estimated 5- and 10-year survival was 48% (95% confidence interval [CI], 36% to 60%) and 29% (95% CI, 16% to 42%), respectively [12]. Three- year survival for patients without lymph node metastases was 69% (95% CI,

Table 1
Incidence of lymph node involvement detected at the time of pulmonary metastasectomy

Authors	Histology	Rate of mediastinal lymph node dissection	Sampling vs lymphadenectomy	Incidence of lymph node metastases
Ercan et al (2004) [12]	Carcinomas	107/883 (12.1%)	Lymphadenectomy	20/70 (28.6%)
Pastorino et al (1997) [2]	Carcinomas & sarcomas	5%	?	239/5206 (4.6%)
Murthy et al (2005) [13]	Renal cell	32/92 (34.8%)	Lymphadenectomy	12/32 (37.5%)
Pfannschmidt et al (2003) [14]	Colorectal	167/167 (100%)	Lymphadenectomy	32/167 (19.1%)
Kamiyoshihara et al (1998) [15]	Carcinomas	22/28 (78.6%)	Lymphadenectomy	6/22 (27.3%)
Loehe et al (2001) [16]	Carcinomas & sarcomas	63/63 (100%)	Lymphadenectomy	9/63 (14.3%)
Pfannschmidt et al (2002) [17]	Renal cell	191/191 (100%)	Lymphadenectomy	57/191 (29.8%)
Inoue et al (2000) [18]	Colorectal	25/25 (100%)	Sampling in 17, lymphadenectomy in 8	7/25 (28%)
Saito et al (2002) [19]	Colorectal	138/165 (83.6%)	Both	20/138 (14.5%)
Okumura et al (1996) [20]	Colorectal	100/159 (62.9%)	Both	15/100 (15%)

Table 2
Lymph node involvement at the time of pulmonary metastasectomy and associated survival

Authors	Histology	5-year survival		P
		Negative nodes	Positive nodes	
Ercan et al (2004) [12]	Carcinomas	68% (at 3 years)	38% (at 3 years)	P < 0.001
Pfannschmidt et al (2003) [14]	Colorectal	38.7%	0%	P < 0.03
Kamiyoshihara et al (1998) [15]	Carcinomas	24.7%	0%	NS
Pfannschmidt et al (2002) [17]	Renal cell	42%	24%	P = 0.016
Inoue et al (2000) [18]	Colorectal	49.5%	14.3%	P = 0.003
Saito et al (2002) [19]	Colorectal	48.5% (at 4 years)	6.2% (at 4 years)	P < 0.001
Okumura et al (1996) [20]	Colorectal	50%	6.7%	P = 0.0004
Piltz et al (2002) [21]	Renal cell	48%	0%	P < 0.001

58% to 83%) as compared with only 38% (95% CI, 20% to 68%) for those with lymph node metastases (P < 0.001) (Fig. 1).

Pfannschmidt and colleagues found that in patients with colorectal primaries, median survival after PM in patients with hilar lymph node metastases alone was 21 months versus 15 months for patients in whom mediastinal lymph nodes were involved [14]. A report from the same authors on patients undergoing PM for renal cell cancer showed no survival difference in patients with hilar or mediastinal lymph node involvement [17]. Murthy and colleagues in a recent study demonstrated that in patients having PM for renal cell cancer, an increasing number of metastatically involved lymph nodes was associated with an incremental risk of death [13].

Therapeutic implications

Although pulmonary metastases reflect M1 and thus stage IV disease, it is apparent that not all metastatic disease behaves the same or carries the same prognosis. Various prognostic indicators may define the biological nature of metastases, predict postresection survival, and assist the clinician in selecting patients who will benefit from surgery. However, no single criterion in patients with respectable pulmo-

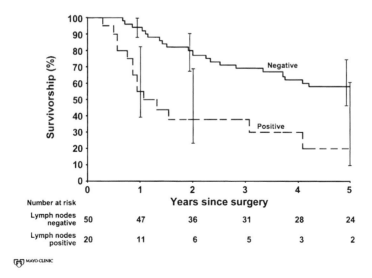

Fig. 1. Estimated survival of 70 patients undergoing pulmonary metastasectomy and complete mediastinal lymphadenectomy without metastatic lymph node involvement (negative) and with lymph node involvement (positive). Zero time on the abscissa is date of first pulmonary metastasectomy and lymph node dissection (P < 0.001). (*From* Ercan S, Nichols III FC, Trastek VF, et al. Prognostic significance of lymph node metastasis found during pulmonary metastasectomy for extrapulmonary carcinoma. Ann Thorac Surg 2004;77:1788; with permission.)

nary metastases consistently and reliably predicts which patients will have long-term survival [4]. Complete resection of pulmonary metastases remains the key characteristic associated with long-term survival.

There appears to be little doubt that the identification of metastatically involved lymph nodes during PM portends a worse prognosis.

Should mediastinal lymphadenectomy be performed in every patient undergoing PM? Arguments favoring such an approach include:

a) There is an incidence of lymph node metastases of 15% to 30%.
b) Chest computerized tomography (CT) has shown a 56% false-negative rate in the evaluation of mediastinal lymph nodes before pulmonary metastasectomy [14].
c) The fact that radiographically detected mediastinal lymphadenopathy did not correlate with lymph node involvement [13].
d) Even patients with only one single pulmonary metastasis can have metastatically involved lymph nodes.
e) Mediastinal lymphadenectomy has a recognized low mortality and morbidity [22].

Positron emission tomography (PET) can be used as a staging modality in patients being considered for PM. In an article by Pastorino and colleagues, PET was able to detect mediastinal lymph node involvement, which was eventually histologically confirmed in seven patients out of 50 undergoing PM [23]. Both the sensitivity and negative predictive value were 100%. However, because the positive predictive value was only 78%, tissue confirmation is still necessary if the patient is to be offered a non-surgical approach.

Whether mediastinal lymphadenectomy during PM has a positive therapeutic effect is unknown. Anecdotally, one of the very first radical lobectomies with lymph node dissection performed at Memorial Sloan-Kettering in 1952 for pulmonary metastases contained metastatically involved lymph nodes. That patient went on to live for 22 years without evidence of recurrence [10]. Although we do not know if mediastinal lymphadenectomy during PM can improve survival, it is likely that unless all metastatically involved lymph nodes are removed, any attempt at cure by resection of pulmonary metastases might be rendered useless.

The clinical impact of metastatic lymph node involvement found during PM remains unknown. There have been no clinical trials demonstrating the results of adjuvant chemotherapy in such patients. Whether novel therapies such as the regional delivery of chemotherapy agents to the lungs, regional hyperthermia, or inhalational therapies might benefit these patients remains to be determined.

Summary

Although surgery for pulmonary metastases does not benefit a significant number of patients, PM should continue to be offered to patients whose primary tumor is controlled and who have acceptable operative risks. For a survival benefit to be achieved, all extrathoracic and pulmonary metastases must be amenable to complete surgical resection. We have shown that the presence of metastatically involved lymph nodes discovered during PM adversely effects survival in patients undergoing curative PM. We therefore continue to recommend complete mediastinal lymphadenectomy at the time of PM to define the patient's prognosis and perhaps to guide adjuvant therapy.

References

[1] Weinlechner JW. Tumoren an der Brustwand und deren Behandlung (Resektion der Rippen, Eronffnung der Brusthoehle, partielle Entfernung der Lunge). Wien Med Wochenschr 1882;32:589–91, 624–8.

[2] Pastorino U, Buyse M, Friedel G, et al. Long-term results of lung metastasectomy: prognostic analyses based an 5206 cases. J Thorac Cardiovasc Surg 1997; 113:37–49.

[3] Martini N, McCormack PM. Evolution of the surgical management of pulmonary metastases. Chest Surg Clin N Am 1998;8:13–27.

[4] Putnam JB. Secondary tumors of the lung. In: Shields TW, LoCicero J, Ponn RB, et al, editors. General Thoracic Surgery. 6th edition. Philadelphia: Lippincott Williams & Wilkins; 2005. p. 1831–62.

[5] Ponn RB, LoCicero J, Daly BD. Surgical treatment of non-small cell lung cancer. In: Shields TW, LoCicero J, Ponn RB, et al, editors. General Thoracic Surgery. 6th edition. Philadelphia: Lippincott Williams & Wilkins; 2005. p. 1548–87.

[6] Rusch VW. Surgical techniques for pulmonary metastasectomy. Semin Thorac Cardiovasc Surg 2002;14: 4–9.

[7] Putnam Jr JB, Roth JA. Prognostic indicators in patients with pulmonary metastases. Semin Surg Oncol 1990;6:291–6.

[8] Pass HI, Donington JS. Metastatic cancer of the lung. In: DeVita V, Hellman S, Rosenberg SA, editors. Principles and Practice of Oncology. Philadelphia: J.B. Lippincott; 1997. p. 2536–51.

[9] Abrams HL, Spiro R, Goldstein N. Metastases in carcinoma: analysis of 1000 autopsied cases. Cancer 1950; 3:75–85.

[10] Thomford NR, Woolner LB, Clagett T. The surgical treatment of metastatic tumors in the lung. J Thorac Cardiovasc Surg 1965;49:357–63.

[11] Cahan WG, Gastro EB, Hajdu SI. Therapeutic pulmonary resection of colonic carcinoma metastatic to lung. Dis Colon Rectum 1974;17:302–9.

[12] Ercan S, Nichols III FC, Trastek VF, et al. Prognostic significance of lymph node metastasis found during pulmonary metastasectomy for extrapulmonary carcinoma. Ann Thorac Surg 2004;77:1786–91.

[13] Murthy SC, Kwhanmien K, Rice TW, et al. Can we predict long-term survival after pulmonary metastasectomy for renal cell carcinoma? Ann Thorac Surg 2005;79:996–1003.

[14] Pfannschmidt J, Muley T, Hoffman H, et al. Prognostic factors and survival after complete resection of pulmonary metastases from colorectal carcinoma: experiences in 167 patients. J Thorac Cardiovasc Surg 2003; 126:732–9.

[15] Kamiyoshihara M, Hirai T, Kawashima O, et al. The surgical treatment of metastatic tumors in the lung: Is lobectomy with mediastinal lymph node dissection suitable treatment? Oncol Rep 1998;5:453–7.

[16] Loehe F, Kobinger S, Hatz RA, et al. Value of systematic mediastinal lymph node dissection during pulmonary metastasectomy. Ann Thorac Surg 2001;72: 225–9.

[17] Pfannschmidt J, Hoffman H, Muley T, et al. Prognostic factors for survival after pulmonary resection of metastatic renal cell carcinoma. Ann Thorac Surg 2002; 74:1653–7.

[18] Inoue M, Kotake Y, Nakagawa K, et al. Surgery for pulmonary metastases from colorectal carcinoma. Ann Thorac Surg 2000;70:380–3.

[19] Saito Y, Omiya H, Kohno K, et al. Pulmonary metastasectomy for 165 patients with colorectal carcinoma: a prognostic assessment. J Thorac Cardiovasc Surg 2002;124:1007–13.

[20] Okumura S, Kondo H, Tsuboi M, et al. Pulmonary resection for metastatic colorectal cancer: experiences with 159 patients. J Thorac Cardiovasc Surg 1996;112: 867–74.

[21] Piltz S, Meimarakis G, Wichmann MW, et al. Long-term results after pulmonary resection of renal cell carcinoma metastases. Ann Thorac Surg 2002;73: 1082–7.

[22] Allen MS, Darling G, Mitchell JD, Z0030 Study Group. Morbidity and mortality of major pulmonary resections in patients with early stage lung cancer: initial results of the randomized prospective ACOSOG Z0030 trial [abstract 3]. Presented at the 41st Annual Meeting of the Society of Thoracic Surgeons. Tampa, January 24–26, 2005.

[23] Pastorino U, Veronesi G, Landoni C, et al. Fluorodeoxyglucose positron emission tomography improves preoperative staging of resectable lung metastasis. J Thorac Cardiovasc Surg 2003;126:1906–10.

ELSEVIER SAUNDERS

Thorac Surg Clin 16 (2006) 145 – 155

THORACIC SURGERY CLINICS

Combined Resection of Liver and Lung Metastases for Colorectal Cancer

Itzhak Avital, MD*, Ronald DeMatteo, MD

Hepatobiliary Service, Department of Surgery, Memorial Sloan-Kettering Cancer Center, 1275 York Avenue, New York, NY 10021, USA

Colon cancer accounts for 10% of all new cancer diagnoses and 11% of all deaths. Across the world, it is the fourth most common malignancy, with approximately one million new cases, and leads to 500,000 deaths each year [1]. In the United States, one in 17 people will have colorectal cancer [2], for an annual incidence that exceeds 145,000 diagnoses. This year, 56,000 Americans will die because of colorectal cancer, making it the second most common cause of cancer death [3].

The liver is the most frequent site of distant metastases in patients with colorectal cancer. Conversely, colorectal cancer is the most common metastatic disease affecting the liver. It is estimated that as many as 25% of patients with colorectal cancer will present with liver metastases when first diagnosed, and another 50% will have hepatic metastases in the ensuing 5 years [4]. Most metachronous metastases occur within 2 years of resection of the primary tumor [5], one-third will have metastases isolated to the liver and of these half will be amenable to resection.

The survival of patients with untreated stage IV colorectal cancer is poor, with a median survival of only 6 to 10 months [6]. Before 2000 [7], systemic chemotherapy improved the outlook for patients with stage IV disease only slightly, leading to a median survival of approximately 12 months [8]. When compared with results achieved by the best chemotherapy available at that time, the value of resection of meta-

static disease in selected patients was clear, as demonstrated by Scheele [9]. Over the past 5 years, new chemotherapeutic agents have improved response rates to more than 50% and the median survival for medically treated patients to more than 20 months [10]. For some investigators, this success has provided a greater impetus for combined modality therapy that includes partial hepatectomy. To others, these new chemotherapeutic regimens and biologic agents have raised questions about the merit of surgery for colorectal metastases.

Elective liver resection for malignancy was first described in the late 19th century [11]. In the last decade, hepatic resection for isolated colorectal liver metastases has become a well-accepted treatment modality [12]. It is reported that liver resection for colorectal metastases provides 5-year survival rates of 20% to 45%, with acceptable rates of perioperative morbidity and minimal perioperative mortality [13].

The lung is the most common extra-abdominal site of metastasis from colorectal carcinoma and approximately 30% of patients with colorectal cancer diagnosed have pulmonary metastases [14,15]. In the past, lung involvement in colorectal cancer was considered as a marker of widespread systemic disease and therefore surgical therapy was felt to be of dubious benefit. Alfred Blalock reported the first successful resection of a pulmonary metastasis from colorectal carcinoma in 1944 [16]. However, it took more than 20 years to establish criteria for resection of pulmonary metastases from colorectal cancer. Thomford, Woolner, and Clagett proposed guidelines in 1965 [17], and these have been updated by Inoue [18]. Although there has never been a prospective

* Corresponding author.

E-mail address: avitali@mskcc.org (I. Avital).

1547-4127/06/$ – see front matter © 2006 Elsevier Inc. All rights reserved.
doi:10.1016/j.thorsurg.2005.12.002

study of the efficacy of pulmonary metastasectomy, it is likely that in at least the highly selected group of patients with long disease-free intervals, and limited number of pulmonary metastases, surgery is beneficial [18]. Patients with lung metastases from colorectal cancer who undergo resection have a 5-year survival of 21% to 43% and a 10-year survival of 20% [18–20].

Approximately 5% to 10% of patients with colorectal cancer will have both liver and pulmonary metastases [21]. The initially poor results seen with chemotherapy alone, together with the encouraging results achieved by metastasectomy of isolated liver or lung metastases, lead to consideration of a more aggressive surgical approach to these patients. The initial reports of combined resection of both hepatic and pulmonary disease sites have been encouraging but are limited by being retrospective and the inclusion of only a small number of patients. Identifying candidates who are most likely to benefit from surgery remains controversial. Therefore, this article evaluates the available evidence for the efficacy of combined liver and lung metastasectomy, and for selection criteria identifying patients most likely to benefit from this approach.

Patients

Between 1998 and 2001, a total of 259 patients were reported in 5 different studies each with [mt]30 patients, demonstrating improved survival after either staged or simultaneous resection of colorectal metastases to the liver and lung (Table 1) [22–26]. These patients included 106 females (40%) and 153 males (60%) with a mean age of 58 years at the time of initial diagnosis of colorectal cancer. The median follow-up ranged from 3.7 to 5.2 years, although the median follow-up was not reported by three of five studies (studies 3–5).

Timing of disease occurrence

Synchronous disease has been defined as metastasis found either at the time of primary tumor diagnosis or within 1 to 3 months of primary tumor resection. The timing of disease presentation was similar among these five studies. Overall, the incidence of synchronous metastatic disease was 18% (47 patients, range in individual studies 0% to 33%). Only one study separated patients with synchronous lung from those with synchronous liver disease [26].

Table 1
Studies reporting combined lung and liver resection for colorectal metastases that include at least 30 patients

Author/ institution	Year	Number of patients	Follow-up (median)	5-year[b] survival
DeMatteo MSKCC	1999	81	3.7 years[a]	38%
Headrick Mayo Clinic	2001	58	5.2 years	30%
Kobayashi[c] Japan	1999	47	NR	31%
Regnard[c] Paris	1998	43	NR	11%
Murata Tokyo	1998	30	NR	44%

NR, not reported.
[a] From time of resection of the first metastasis.
[b] Once both liver and lung resection performed.
[c] Multicenter study.

In this study, 75% of synchronous metastases involved the liver, whereas 25% had combined liver and lung disease. Curiously, none of these studies reported the incidence of isolated synchronous lung metastases (Fig. 1).

The time to first diagnosis of metachronous disease (first disease-free interval [DFI-1]) was strikingly similar among the various studies at a median of 1.0 to 1.3 years (range, 0 to 15 years). Two studies (studies 3 and 5) did not report on time to first recurrence. The majority of first recurrences were in the liver 62% (160 patients). Simultaneous (liver and lung) first recurrences were more common than lung alone as a first recurrence (17% or 45 patients versus 3% or 13 patients, respectively). Only one study (study 1) reported on the prevalence of patients with a DFI-1 of less than 1 year, which occurred in 46% or 37 patients.

The interval between the first recurrence after primary tumor diagnosis and the second recurrence (second disease-free interval [DFI-2]) was again similar across these five studies, although somewhat more variable than DFI-1. The most common site for secondary recurrence was the lung, which occurred with a median of 1.2 to 3.2 years (0 to 8.5 years) after first metastasectomy. Only one study (study 1) reported on the prevalence of DFI-2 of less than 1 year, which occurred in 47% or 38 patients. It appears that in these studies, approximately 50% of the patients recurred within 1 year of the first liver metastasectomy.

Two studies reported on concurrent other metastases; however, the exact timing of their occurrence is not noted. Study 1 reported on bone (7%), lymph nodes (7%), and brain (1.2%) metastases, whereas

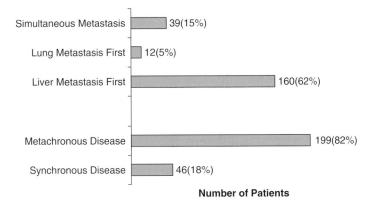

Fig. 1. Temporal relationships of colorectal metastases.

study 5 reported on abdominal wall (3.3%) and lymph node (6.6%) metastases.

Clinicopathologic features of the primary colon cancer

Among 201 reported cases, 65% (131 patients) and 35% (70 patients) had their primary disease in the colon and rectum, respectively (Table 2). Four

patients (2%) were not characterized. Study 2 did not distinguish among the various sites of the primary colorectal cancer.

The reporting of stage was variable in the five studies we analyzed. Study 3 did not report the stage of the primary tumor at all, whereas only study 2 used the TNM system. Among the patients who were staged according to the TNM system, 0% had stage I, 35% (20 patients) had stage II, 41% (24 patients) had stage III, and 22% (13 patients) had stage IV. Of the remaining 151 patients, 3% (4 patients) had Duke's A,

Table 2
Clinicopathologic features of the primary colon cancer

Study/ institution	Primary tumor		Stage (Dukes/TNM)		Synchronous disease	Histology		Age (years)	Sex	
DeMatteo MSKCC	Colon Rectum	62 19	A B C D	2 (3%) 21 (27%) 32 (40%) 24 (30%)	24 (30%)	47 (59%) patients had positive nodes		59	Female Male	32 49
Headrick Mayo Clinic	NR		I II III IV	0 20 (35%) 24 (41%) 13 (22%)	4 (7%)	Grade II Grade III	48% 29%	59	Female Male	21 37
Kobayashi[a] Japan	Colon Rectum NR	26 17 4	NR		7 (15%)	NR		59	Female Male	17 30
Regnard[a] Paris	Colon Rectum	28 19	A B C D	0 7 22 14	NR	WD UD CC	39 2 2	54	Female Male	18 25
Murata Tokyo	Colon Rectum	15 15	A B C D	2 (6%) 4 (1.5%) 13 (43%) 10 (33%)	10 (33%)	NR		59	Female Male	18 12

Abbreviations: CC, colloid carcinoma; UD, undifferentiated; WD, well-differentiated.
[a] Multi-center study.

Table 3
Clinicopathologic features of the lung metastases

Study	Number of lesions		Distribution		Size (cm)		Lymph node involvement	Surgical procedures	
DeMatteo MSKCC	1	38 (51%)	Unilateral	65 (81%)	≤2	60 (81%)	NR	Wedge	68 (84%)
	>1	37 (49%)	Bilateral	15 (19%)	>2	14 (19%)		Lobe	13 (16%)
Headrick Mayo Clinic	1	31 (53%)	NR		NR		N1 2(3.5%)	Wedge	20 (52%)
	2	13 (22%)					N2 2(3.5%)	Lobe	6 (10%)
	3	10 (17%)						Multiple	22 (38%)
	4	4 (7%)						Wedge	
Kobayashi[a] Metastatic Lung Tumor Study Group of Japan	1	21 (45%)	Unilateral	38 (80%)	<2	19 (40%)	NR	Wedge	18 (38%)
	1–3	17 (36%)	Bilateral	9 (19%)	2–2.9	11 (23%)		Lobe	15 (32%)
	4–5	5 (10%)			3–4.9	12 (26%)		Segment	14 (30%)
	≥6	4 (9.0%)			≥5	2 (5%)			
Regnard[a] Institut Mutualiste Montsouris, Paris, France	1	(2–12)	NR		NR		N2 6(14%)	Wedge	6 (14%)
	(median)							Lobe	5 (12%)
								Segment	3 (7%)
								Pneumonectomy	2 (5%)
								Tumorectomy	27 (65%)
Murata National Cancer Center Tokyo, Japan	1	18 (60%)	Unilateral	25 (83%)	≤3	23 (76%)	6 (20%)[b]	Wedge	9 (30%)
	2	5 (16%)	Bilateral	5 (16%)	>3	7 (23%)		Lobe & segment	15 (50%)
	3	3 (10%)						Both	6 (20%)
	4	2 (6%)							
	>4	2 (6%)							

[a] Multicenter study.
[b] Lymphatic and vascular invasion.

21% (32 patients) had Duke's B, 44% (67 patients) had Duke's C, and 32% (48 patients) had Duke's D. Thus, the majority of the patients had nodal involvement and/or distant metastases at presentation.

Interestingly, only limited information regarding histopathology was reported. Study 2 reported that 48% and 29% of their cohort had a grade II and grade III colorectal cancer, respectively. Study 4 provided information on the degree of differentiation. Well-differentiated colorectal cancer was the most common and seen in 90% (39 patients), whereas undifferentiated and colloid carcinoma were rare (5% or 2 patients each).

Clinicopathologic features of the liver metastases

In all, 61% (146 patients) had solitary lesions and 39% (90 patients) had more than one metastatic lesion (Table 3). Studies 2 and 3 further specified the number of lesions in 95 patients: 22% (21 patients) had two lesions, 5% (5 patients) had three lesions, and 6% (6 patients) had four lesions. The median number of lesions was one. The most common intrahepatic distribution was unilateral 70% (105 patients) (2 studies did not report distribution). Only studies 1 and 5 reported the size of the lesions. The size of the lesions was under-reported because it was stated only

in studies 1 and 5. There were 46 patients (45% of 104 patients) with lesions 5 cm or smaller, 47 patients (45%) with lesions 4 to 5 cm, and 11 patients with lesions larger than 5 cm (10%); 77 (30%) patients underwent hepatic wedge resections, 30 (12%) had segmentectomy, 63 (25%) had lobectomy, 47 (18%) had extended lobectomy, 44 (17%) had anatomic resections (segmentectomy or lobectomy), and seven (3%) underwent multiple simultaneous resections. Study 1 reported 10 patients who had hepatic arterial pumps placed at the time of liver resection.

Clinicopathologic features of the lung metastases

The features of the lung metastases are listed in Table 4. The median number of lung lesions was reported in studies 1 and 4 as being one lesion (range, 1–14). In addition, among 216 reported patients, only 108 (50%) had a single lesion. However, three studies reported on resection of multiple (≥4) lung metastases. Of these 135 reported patients, 17 (13%) had four or more lesions resected.

The majority of the patients had lesions localized to one lung. Studies 1, 3, and 5 reported on the distribution of the lesions in 158 patients. In this group, 128 (81%) had unilateral disease, and most (65%) of these lesions were smaller than 2 cm. Large

Table 4
Clinicopathologic features of the liver metastases

Study	Number of lesions		Distribution		Size (cm)		Surgical procedures		Pump
DeMatteo	1	41 (58%)	Unilateral	48 (62%)	≤4	27 (36%)	Wedge	12 (15%)	10 (12%)
MSKCC	>1	30 (42%)	Bilateral	29 (38%)	>4	47 (64%)	Segment	18 (22%)	
	Median 1 (1–8)				Median 4.5		Lobectomy	27 (33%)	
					(1.5–20)				
							Extended Lobectomy	24 (30%)	
Headrick	1	30 (57%)	NR		NR		Wedge	25 (43%)	NR
Mayo	2	10 (17%)					Lobectomy	12 (21%)	
Clinic	3	3 (5%)					Extended Lobectomy	20 (34%)	
	4	2 (3%)					Multiple Wedge	1 (2%)	
Kobayashi[a]	1	30 (63%)	NR		NR		Wedge	15 (32%)	NR
Japan	2	11 (23%)					Segment	12 (25%)	
	3	2 (6%)					Bi-segment	2 (4%)	
	4	4 (8%)					Lobectomy	16 (34%)	
Regnard[a]	1	25 (58%)	Unilateral	36 (84%)	NR		Wedge	10 (23%)	NR
Paris	>1	18 (42%)	Bilateral	7 (16%)			Anatomic Resections	33 (77%)	
Murata	1	20 (66%)	Unilateral	21 (70%)	≤5	19 (63%)	Wedge	15 (50%)	NR
Tokyo	>1	10 (33%)	Bilateral	9 (30%)	>5	11 (36%)	Anatomic Resections	11 (36%)	
							Both	4 (13%)	

[a] Multi-center study.

($\geq$5cm) lesions were resected in nine (6%) patients. Nodal involvement in the chest was reported by studies 2, 4, and 5. Of these 131 patients, 16 (12%) had nodal involvement, with eight (50%) having N2 disease. The most common thoracic procedure reported was wedge resection or segmentectomy in 165 (63%) patients. Lobectomy was required by 39 (15%) patients, and 45 (17%) patients underwent multiple procedures (ie, multiple wedges or lobectomy plus another procedure). Pneumonectomy was performed in only two (0.6%) patients.

Complications

Minimal data regarding complications were provided by these studies. Studies 1 and 3 did not report on their complication rate. Interestingly, in the studies that did report complications (studies 2, 4, and 5) the mortality was 0%. Morbidity ranged between 5% and 12%, which is lower than most other studies reporting on colorectal cancer metastatic to the liver or lung. The most common complications reported were bowel obstruction, postoperative hemorrhage, bile leak, chyle leak, empyema, and pulmonary embolus. Complication grade could be assessed in only studies 4 and 5, and only three (4%) patients had grade 3 complications, which is defined as a complication that requires an invasive intervention [27].

Neoadjuvant and adjuvant therapy

Neoadjuvant therapy for the primary colorectal lesion was not reported among these studies, even though they reported on rectal lesions. Studies 1, 2, and 4 reported in adequate detail on adjuvant chemoradiotherapy after resection of the primary colorectal lesion. Of 169 patients, 67(40%) received chemotherapy, 6 (4%) radiation therapy, and 19 (11%) had both chemotherapy and radiation therapy.

In recent years, neoadjuvant chemotherapy has been explored in an attempt to render more patients candidates for resection of metastases [28]. Therefore, it is interesting that only one study [25] reported on neoadjuvant therapy before liver or lung metastasectomy. In this study, 15 (35%) patients received chemotherapy only before lung metastasectomy. Studies 2, 4, and 5 reported on adjuvant therapy after metastasectomy. Of 131 patients, 22 (17%) received adjuvant chemotherapy after liver resection alone,

41 (31%) after lung metastasectomy, two (1.5%) after both liver and colon resection, and one patient after both the lung and the liver metastasectomy.

Recurrence

Local recurrence after resection of the primary colorectal lesion was similar between the reporting studies [23,25,26]. Of 154 reported patients, 16 (10%) had local recurrences. Recurrences after the first metastasectomy were reported by studies 1, 4, and 5. The incidence of any recurrence after first metastasectomy ranged between 11% and 23%. Study 5 reported on organ-specific recurrences, noting that 17 patients had their first metastases in the liver and three recurred; one whose recurrence was in the lung and two with recurrence in both lung and liver.

Recurrences after a second metastasectomy were approximately three times as frequent as after the first metastasectomy. Of 201 patients, 58 (29%) had recurrence after the second metastasectomy. The incidence varied widely among these studies. The lowest recurrence rate was 12% as reported by study 3. The highest recurrence rate was reported by study 5. In this series, among 30 patients, 43% had recurrence in the liver, 50% in the lung, and 26% in other loci (brain, bone, lymph nodes, and peritoneal cavity). Study 1 reported on patients with tertiary recurrences who underwent resection. Of 81 patients, four (5%) had recurrence after the second metastasectomy, which had required lung resection.

Survival

Survival analysis differed between the five studies. Studies 1 and 5 measured survival from the time of resection of the primary lesion. The median survival in these patients ranged from 4 (0.9–12.5) to 8.2 (0.6 – 14.3) years. Further, study 1 reported that the 1-, 3-, and 5-year actuarial survival after resection of the colon was 96%, 77%, and 58%, respectively (Table 5).

Median survival after first metastasectomy was also reported by study 1 as being 6 years. The median survival after both the liver and the lung resections had been performed was reported by studies 1, 4, and 5 as ranging between 1.6 and 3.8 years. Study 1 reported on actuarial survival after resection of the colon: 1-year survival was 96%, 3-year survival was 77%, and 5-year survival was 58% (Table 5).

Table 5
Survival[b]

Study	From primary colon (median/years)	From first metastasis (median/years)	After liver and lung resection (median/years)	Actuarial survival from colon resection		Actuarial survival after lung and liver resection (years)	
DeMatteo MSKCC	8.2 (0.6–14.3)	6.0 (0.08–13.5)	3.8 (0.08–10.8)	1 year	96%	1	93%
				3 years	77%	3	62%
				5 years	58%	5	38%
						Number from first metastasectomy	
						5	40%
Headrick Mayo Clinic	NR	NR	NR	NR		5	30%
						10	16%
						(After first lung resection)	
Kobayashi[a] Japan	NR	NR	NR	NR		3	36%
						5	31%
						8	23%
Regnard[a] Paris	NR	NR	1.6 (6–72)	NR		5 years	11%
Murata Tokyo	4 (0.9–12.5)	NR	2.5 (0.6–8.5)	NR		1	86.7%
						3	49.3%
						5	43.8%

[a] Multicenter study.
[b] Disease-specific survival.

All studies reported various periods of actuarial survival. The most commonly reported period of actuarial survival was that after both liver and lung metastasectomy, which ranged from 11% to 44% at 5 years. One-year survival was reported by two studies (111 patients) and ranged between 87% and 93%. Three-year survival was reported by three studies (158 patients) and ranged between 36% and 62%. Study 2 reported a 10-year actuarial survival of 16% after lung resection.

Four studies reported that the percentage of patients who were disease-free ranged from 12% to 40%. Study 1 reported on the actual number of patients surviving 3, 5, and 10 years: 50 (62%) patients, 24 (30%), and three (12%), respectively. Patients who had simultaneous metastases (liver and lung) had worse outcome than patients with metachronous metastasis. Survival in patients who had simultaneous metastatic disease in the liver and lung was 22% at 5 years with a median survival of 2 (0.75 – 5.2) years, whereas survival of patients who had metachronous metastases was 50% to 58% at 5 years with a median survival of 2.6 (0.6-9) years [23,24].

Survival was analyzed based on the features of the pulmonary metastasis in study 3. Survival of patients with a single metastasis was superior to those with multiple lung metastases. Survival of patients with solitary lung lesions at 3, 5, and 8 years was 48%, 40% and 40%, respectively. In contrast, survival of patients with multiple lung lesions at 3, 5, and 8 years was 30%, 22%, and 0%, respectively. Interestingly,

in this study no patient with multiple lung metastases survived 8 years. The extent of resection influenced survival. The 5-year survival of patients undergoing pulmonary wedge or segmentectomy versus lobectomy was 22% and 44%, respectively.

Prognostic factors

Prognostic factors for survival in these studies are shown in Table 6. Notably, the statistical methods used to analyze these factors differed between these studies.

Overall, 23 factors were analyzed in the following categories: demographics (age and gender), primary tumor characteristics (site, nodal involvement, and adjuvant therapy), liver metastases (number, size, laterality, type of resection, timing of resection, and bile duct invasion), lung metastases (number, size, laterality, type of resection, thoracic lymph node involvement, and timing of resection), timing of metastases (synchronous, simultaneous [liver and lung at the same time], metachronous, DFI-1, and DFI-2), and CEA. Table 7 lists factors that were not found to predict survival (Table 7).

By univariate analysis, lung involvement as the first site of metastasis ($P < 0.004$), [26] normal CEA ($P < 0.03$) [22,25] unilateral lung metastasis ($P < 0.04$), [24] and simultaneous liver–lung metastases ($P < 0.009$) [24] were important predictors of outcome. Different studies found different variables

Table 6
Prognostic factors (multivariate analysis)

Study	DFI-2	CEA[b]	Number of lung nodules	Lung resection	Distribution of lung metastases	Other	Trends
DeMatteo MSKCC	DFI-2 >1 year[a]	NR	No	NR	No	No	Improved survival with adjuvant chemotherapy after primary colon disease
Headrick Mayo Clinic	No	5 ng/mL	No	No	NR	Decreased survival with N2 lung disease	Decreased survival with shorter disease-free interval
Kobayashi[a] Japan	Synchronous vs metachronous liver before lung	NR	Solitary pulmonary metastases (after last metastasectomy)	No	NR	Longer DFI-2 (after first metastasectomy)	90% of patients who survived >3 years had ≤2 liver metastases
Regnard[a] Paris	DFI-2 >3 year[a]	5 ng/mL	No	One vs > one procedure	No	N2 lung disease did not predict poor survival	
Murata Tokyo	Synchronous vs metachronous	NR	No	No	Unilateral vs bilateral		

[a] DFI-2: disease-free interval between first and second metastases.
[b] CEA before metastasectomy.

Table 7
Prognostic factors significant by multivariate analysis

Factors that did not achieve significance common to all
five studies reporting on more than 30 patients

Age	Grade of primary tumor
Gender	Number of hepatic metastases
Colon vs rectum	Diameter of metastases
Nodal status	Method of pulmonary resection
Adjuvant therapy for the primary lesion	Method of hepatic resection

to be significant on multivariate analysis. Multivariate analysis revealed that the following factors were found to be statistically significant in at least one study: DFI-2, synchronous disease, liver metastasis before lung metastasis, CEA level less than 5 ng/mL, solitary lung metastasis, multiple pulmonary resections, unilateral lung disease, and thoracic nodal involvement. DFI-2 was reported in four of the studies and was important [23–26]. The chances for survival are better the longer the interval between the first metastasis and the second metastasis for patients with metachronous disease.

Prognostic factors reported in less than three of the studies that were found to be statistically significant were synchronous disease [23,24] and CEA level (<5 ng/mL) [22,25], solitary lung metastases by 20% [24], liver metastasis before lung metastasis [24], and unilateral pulmonary disease [23].

Interestingly, several factors were reported as trending toward but not reaching statistical significance. The only factor regarding liver disease which was reported to impact survival was the fact that 90% of the patients who survived more than 3 years had two or fewer liver metastases [24]. Additionally, improved survival was more common in patients who received adjuvant therapy after resection of the primary colon lesion [26]. Given the small numbers of patients in these studies, these factors may be worth considering for evaluation in larger trials.

Among the factors that were found to be statistically significant on multivariate analysis, only one was inconsistent. Study 2 found that N2 lung disease was associated with decreased survival, whereas study 4 found that N2 lung disease did not predict poor survival.

Discussion

Resection of isolated hepatic or pulmonary metastases from colorectal cancer has been shown to be safe and probably beneficial. Improvements in the understanding of anatomy, perioperative care, and surgical technique have reduced the operative mortality for liver resection to less than 5%, and for most pulmonary metastasectomies to less than 1% [9,13]. In our recent experience of 1001 patients who underwent hepatectomy for colorectal metastases [29], the 5-year survival was 37%. Similarly, in a series of 144 patients who had pulmonary resection for colorectal metastases at our institution, the 5- and 10-year survival rates were 40% and 30%, respectively [30]. Even if the resection of isolated liver or lung metastases from colorectal cancer is beneficial, the benefit of surgery in patients with both liver and lung metastases either simultaneously or metachronously is not well-defined. It is surprising that there are so few studies of combined liver and lung metastasectomy for colorectal cancer that either report on more than 30 patients, or have been published recently (4 of the 5 reports date to before 2000). Study 5 reported that 30 patients who underwent combined liver and lung metastasectomy had a 5-year survival of 44%, and we reported on 38% survival at 5 years (n=81) with a median follow-up of 3.7 years. The longest follow-up of a median of 5.2 years was reported by study 2. In this population the survival was 30% at 5 years. In contrast, study 4 reported an 11% survival at 5 years (n=43). It is likely that with the recent developments in chemotherapy and biologic agents, outcome will be further improved.

Patient selection is obviously critical when considering resection of liver and lung metastases from colorectal cancer. It should be noted that the majority of the reported patients had favorable metastatic disease (single liver and lung metastases). Previously, we developed a 5-point scoring after hepatectomy for colorectal metastases [29]. Applying these criteria to the five studies discussed in this chapter, 61% of the patients had solitary liver metastasis, 50% had liver metastases less than 5 cm, fewer than 50% of the patients had nodal disease, and the median time to first recurrence was more than 1 year. Therefore, it seems that on balance, more than 50% of the patients in these studies had a favorable (ie, <3 points) clinical risk score. This scoring system may be useful in selecting patients for combined liver and lung metastasectomy for colorectal cancer.

There were several predictors of poor outcome in these studies on multivariate analysis. A disease-free interval between the first and the second metastases of less than 1 year [24–26], synchronous disease [23,24], lung metastasis before liver metastasis [24], multiple lung metastases [24], multiple lung resections [25], and bilateral lung involvement [23]. It seems that with the exception of synchronous disease, the characteristics of the secondary recurrence, particularly if the recurrence is pulmonary, have a major impact on survival. It is interesting that none of the liver clinicopathologic parameters affected the outcome of these patients. This may have been because of selection bias, because most of these patients had low score on our prognostic index. Alternatively, the biology of lung metastases may override the influence of liver metastases in this group of patients.

In these studies, the majority of patients received 5-FU–based chemotherapy. Presently, the standard of care is FOLFOX of FOLFIRI with or without Avastin and survival has been markedly improved to a median exceeding 20 months [10]. This raises the question of whether surgical resection of colorectal metastases should be continued. However, an argument could be made that, in general, the only chance of cure is through surgical resection in combination with systemic therapy. There is currently no data to support or refute these positions. The use of neoadjuvant therapy may be used to select patients with favorable disease [28].

In conclusion, highly selected patients with both liver and lung metastases should be offered surgical therapy because a 5-year survival rate of 44% can be achieved. Surgery offers the only possibility for prolonged survival and is occasionally curative. The ideal patient would have one or two metachronous liver metastases that occurred more than 1 year after the primary disease and then more than 1 year later would have a single lung recurrence. Studies using the more effective chemotherapeutic regimens in combination with surgery need to be performed.

References

[1] Jemal A, Murray T, Ward E, et al. Cancer statistics, 2005. CA Cancer J Clin 2005;55:10–30.

[2] National Cancer Institute. Statistical Research and Applications Branch. Available at: http://srab.cancer.gov/devcan. Accessed May 15, 2005.

[3] American Cancer Society. Cancer Figures and Facts. Available at: http://cancer.org. Accessed May 15, 2005.

[4] Bengmark S, Hafstrom L. The natural history of primary and secondary malignant tumors of the liver. I. The prognosis for patients with hepatic metastases from colonic and rectal carcinoma by laparotomy. Cancer 1969;23:198–202.

[5] Ridge JA, Daly JM. Treatment of colorectal hepatic metastases. Surg Gynecol Obstet 1985;161:597–607.

[6] Bengmark S, Hafstrom L. The natural history of primary and secondary malignant tumors of the liver. II. The prognosis for patients with hepatic metastases

[7] from gastric carcinoma verified by laparotomy and postmortem examination. Digestion 1969;2:179–86.

[7] de Gramont A, Figer A, Seymour M, et al. Leucovorin and fluorouracil with or without oxaliplatin as first-line treatment in advanced colorectal cancer. J Clin Oncol 2000;18:2938–47.

[8] Cunningham D, Pyrhonen S, James RD, et al. Randomised trial of irinotecan plus supportive care versus supportive care alone after fluorouracil failure for patients with metastatic colorectal cancer. Lancet 1998; 352(9138):1413–8.

[9] Scheele J, Stang R, Altendorf-Hofmann A, et al. Resection of colorectal liver metastases. World J Surg 1995;19:59–71.

[10] Meyerhardt JA, Mayer RJ. Systemic therapy for colorectal cancer. N Engl J Med 2005;352:476–87.

[11] Keen W. Report of a case of resection of the liver for the removal of a neoplasm with a table of seventy six cases of resection of the liver for hepatic tumours. Ann Surg 1889;30:267–83.

[12] Petrowsky H, Gonen M, Jarnagin W, et al. Second liver resections are safe and effective treatment for recurrent hepatic metastases from colorectal cancer: a bi-institutional analysis. Ann Surg 2002;235:863–71.

[13] Fong Y, Cohen AM, Fortner JG, et al. Liver resection for colorectal metastases. J Clin Oncol 1997;15: 938–46.

[14] Gilbert G. sites of recurrent tumour after curative colorectal surgery: implications for adjuvant therapy. Br J Surg 1984;71:203–5.

[15] Welch JP, Donaldson GA. Detection and treatment of recurrent cancer of the colon and rectum. Am J Surg 1978;135:505–11.

[16] Blalock AB. Recent advances in surgery. N Engl J Med 1944;231:261–7.

[17] Thomford NR WL, Clagett OT. The surgical teatment of metastatic tumors in the lung. J Thoracic Cardiovas Surg 1965;49:357–63.

[18] Inoue M, Ohta M, Iuchi K, et al. Benefits of surgery for patients with pulmonary metastases from colorectal carcinoma. Ann Thorac Surg 2004;78:238–44.

[19] Girard P, Ducreux M, Baldeyrou P, et al. Surgery for lung metastases from colorectal cancer: analysis of prognostic factors. J Clin Oncol 1996;14:2047–53.

[20] McAfee MK, Allen MS, Trastek VF, et al. Colorectal lung metastases: results of surgical excision. Ann Thorac Surg 1992;53:780–5 [discussion 785–6].

[21] Pihl E, Hughes ES, McDermott FT, et al. Lung recurrence after curative surgery for colorectal cancer. Dis Colon Rectum 1987;30:417–9.

[22] Headrick JR, Miller DL, Nagorney DM, et al. Surgical treatment of hepatic and pulmonary metastases from colon cancer. Ann Thorac Surg 2001;71:975–9 [discussion 979–80].

[23] Murata S, Moriya Y, Akasu T, et al. Resection of both hepatic and pulmonary metastases in patients with colorectal carcinoma. Cancer 1998;83:1086–93.

[24] Kobayashi K, Kawamura M, Ishihara T. Surgical treatment for both pulmonary and hepatic metastases from

colorectal cancer. J Thorac Cardiovasc Surg 1999;118: 1090–6.

[25] Regnard JF, Grunenwald D, Spaggiari L, et al. Surgical treatment of hepatic and pulmonary metastases from colorectal cancers. Ann Thorac Surg 1998;66:214–8 [discussion 218–9].

[26] DeMatteo RM, Minnard EA, Kemeney N, et al. Surgical resection of both hepatic and pulmonary metastases in patients with colorectal cancer. Proceedings of ASCO 1999. Abstract 958.

[27] Martin 2nd RC, Brennan MF, Jaques DP. Quality of complication reporting in the surgical literature. Ann Surg 2002;235:803–13.

[28] Leonard GD, Brenner B, Kemeny NE. Neoadjuvant chemotherapy before liver resection for patients with unresectable liver metastases from colorectal carcinoma. J Clin Oncol 2005;23:2038–48.

[29] Fong Y, Fortner J, Sun RL, et al. Clinical score for predicting recurrence after hepatic resection for metastatic colorectal cancer: analysis of 1001 consecutive cases. Ann Surg 1999;230:309–18 [discussion 318–21].

[30] McCormack PM, Burt ME, Bains MS, et al. Lung resection for colorectal metastases. 10-year results. Arch Surg 1992;127:1403–6.

ELSEVIER
SAUNDERS

Thorac Surg Clin 16 (2006) 157–165

THORACIC
SURGERY
CLINICS

Minimally Invasive Techniques for Managing Pulmonary Metastases: Video-assisted Thoracic Surgery and Radiofrequency Ablation

Ara Ketchedjian, MD[a], Benedict Daly, MD[a], James Luketich, MD[b], Hiran C. Fernando, MBBS, FRCS[a],*

[a]Department of Cardiothoracic Surgery, Boston Medical Center, 88 East Newton Street, Robinson B-402, Boston, MA 02118-2392, USA
[b]Heart Lung and Esophageal Institute, University of Pittsburgh Medical Center, C-800, PUH, 200 Lothrop Street, Pittsburgh, PA 15213, USA

The survival benefit of pulmonary metastasectomy has been supported by multiple retrospective studies. Patients who are most likely to benefit from surgical intervention are those in who local control of the primary tumor has been or can be achieved, who have experienced a long disease-free interval from primary tumor resection, for who no effective alternative therapy exists, who do not have any extra thoracic metastases, and who have a limited pulmonary metastatic burden that can be completely resected [1]. These principals were illustrated in the largest series of pulmonary metastectomy reported by the International Registry of Lung Metastases [2]. In this series of 5206 cases, 5-year survival was 33% when the disease-free interval was 0 to 11 months compared with 45% for those with a disease-free interval of more than 36 months. Similarly, patients with solitary sites of pulmonary metastatic disease had a survival of 43% compared with 27% for patients with four or more lesions. Thoracotomy with bi-manual palpation has been the standard treatment for metastatic pulmonary disease, because this has been demonstrated to provide the best way of identifying all but micrometastatic disease. In some tumors, such as sarcomas, bilateral thoracotomy or sternotomy has been recommended to look for radiographically occult disease present in the contralateral lung [3]. Although an open approach is felt to optimally identify sites of disease, many centers are increasingly using minimally invasive approaches to treat pulmonary metastases, because of the lower morbidity and the potential to preserve pulmonary and physical function, particularly in patients who are at increased risk for open operations [4]. In this chapter we review the use of video-assisted thoracic surgery (VATS) and radiofrequency ablation (RFA) for pulmonary metastases. The relative benefits and disadvantages of these techniques are discussed to help define when it is appropriate to use either method.

Video-assisted thoracic surgery

Over the past two decades, minimally invasive techniques have revolutionized general and thoracic surgery. In 1992, surgeons at the University of Pittsburgh provided the first report of VATS for pulmonary metastases in a report describing the use of the Nd:YAG laser to resect a solitary renal cell carcinoma metastasis [5]. The next year, the first series of VATS metastasectomy in 72 patients was

* Corresponding author. Department of Cardiothoracic Surgery, 88 East Newton Street, Robinson B-402 Boston, MA 02118-2392.
E-mail address: hiran.fernando@bmc.org (H.C. Fernando).

1547-4127/06/$ – see front matter © 2006 Elsevier Inc. All rights reserved.
doi:10.1016/j.thorsurg.2005.11.002

reported from the same center. The authors concluded that VATS was a feasible operative technique for the treatment of metastatic lung disease and that it reduced overall hospital stay compared with historical controls. In the ensuing years VATS has been used for increasingly more complex thoracic procedures such as esophagomyotomy [6], lobectomy [7], and even esophagectomy [8].

The use of VATS, however, remains controversial for pulmonary metastases. The primary argument against the use of VATS is the lack of the ability to bimanually palpate the lung and completely resect all macroscopic metastases [9]. Several series have shown that when complete resection is performed survival is statistically better [10,11]. In the International Registry of Lung Metastases study of 5206 patients, 5-year survival was 36% for complete resection compared with 13% when resections were incomplete [2].

One of the strongest papers arguing against the use of VATS was the prospective study comparing VATS to thoracotomy by McCormack and colleagues from Memorial Sloan-Kettering Cancer Center [9]. This study with a planned accrual of 50 patients was closed after enrolling only 18 patients because a statistically significant benefit to thoracotomy was found. In 15 (83%) patients, all nodules seen with computed tomography (CT) were identified and resected by VATS. However, when these same patients were explored by thoracotomy, additional malignant nodules were identified in 56% (10/18) patients that were not seen on CT or detected during VATS. The authors concluded that VATS was inadequate for therapy and that its use should be reserved as a diagnostic tool only.

After this trial, it has been argued that VATS for pulmonary metastasectomy should not be performed except for the patient unable to tolerate thoracotomy, or as a diagnostic tool, or perhaps for the patient with single metastasis. Subsequent studies have investigated this problem further. First, a more recent Dutch study used a similar study design in 28 patients explored first by VATS and then by thoracotomy [12]. VATS resection was not possible in 10 patients, and one patient with carcinoid was excluded from the study. Seventeen patients were left for analysis, of whom 12 had a single lesion on preoperative CT scan. The success rate was higher in patients with a single lesion, with 11 of 12 (91.7%) having all disease resected by VATS compared with 1 of 5 (20%) in those who had more than one lesion on CT. This study can be criticized in that 10 patients (35.7%) had an unsuccessful VATS excision [12]. This is higher than the technical failure rates noted in other series

and may have been partly caused by their inclusion of central tumors in this study. Most surgeons would agree that VATS wedge resections for metastases should be reserved for peripheral rather than central lesions.

Mutsaerts and colleagues recently reported on a small study comparing eight patients treated with VATS metastasectomy alone to 12 patients treated with VATS followed by confirmatory thoracotomy [13]. Although the numbers were small, the 2-year overall survivals were at 67% (VATS patients) and 70% (open patients), implying that VATS was safe with similar outcomes as thoracotomy.

The series from Memorial Sloan Kettering used older-generation CT scans, which may have decreased their ability to detect metastases [9]. It has been argued that if helical CT scans had been performed, a greater number of nodules may have been identified before proceeding to thoracotomy. An Italian study retrospectively compared the accuracy of high-resolution CT (HRCT) scan in 78 patients to 88 patients who had helical CT (HCT) scan [14]. All patients subsequently underwent thoracotomy for resection of lung metastases. The sensitivity of the newer-generation HCT scans was better at 82.1% compared with 75% for the HRCT scans, although the results were not statistically significant. For small lesions (defined as 6 mm or less) the sensitivity was worse, at 61.5% and 48% for the HCT and HRCT, respectively. Despite the improved definition seen with the newer generation scanners, it appears that lung nodules, particularly if small, may be missed unless thoracotomy is performed.

One of the primary reasons for using VATS has been the expectation that morbidity will be less and recovery will be faster. Ninomiya and colleagues. compared pulmonary function in patients undergoing metastasectomy by VATS or by thoracotomy [15]. In the VATS group, the early and late decrease in vital capacity was 16.2% and 2.0%, respectively. Both were significantly less than the early (33%) and late (17.7%) decrease in vital capacity after thoracotomy. The authors also compared the decrease in percent vital capacity after reoperative VATS and reoperative thoracotomy for recurrent metastatic disease and found that the decrease was significantly less in the VATS group (21.3%) than in the thoracotomy patients (61%). Landreneau and colleagues. compared postoperative pain and shoulder function after VATS or thoracotomy [4]. Two groups were studied, the first of which included 239 patients less than 1 year from surgery and the second included 104 patients who were at least 1 year out from surgery. In the group that was less than 1 year out from surgery, significantly less pain and shoulder dysfunction was present in the VATS patients. In the group who were at least 1 year out from their operations, no difference was found. In another study by the same investigators, impairment of FEV1% was significantly worse in thoracotomy patients compared with VATS patients having lung resections [16] 1 week after surgery; however, by postoperative week 3, this difference was no longer present.

An unfavorable prognosis is understandable if gross unresectable disease is left behind after surgery. This was certainly the case in studies such as that by the International Registry of Lung Metastases, in which patients with incomplete resections after thoracotomy had significantly poorer survival compared with patients who had complete resections [2]. However, the extent to which the resection of radiologically occult lesions improves survival is unclear. If resection of all disease that can be detected by palpation is important, then it can be argued that bilateral thoracotomies should be routinely performed. Roth and colleagues compared the results of metastasectomy in sarcoma patients undergoing either sternotomy with bimanual palpation of both lungs or thoracotomy of one lung [17]. The groups were matched for the number of nodules, the tumor doubling time, and disease-free interval. Despite 45% of the patients undergoing sternotomy being found to have occult metastases in the contralateral lung, bilateral exploration and resection did not confer a survival benefit. Further, other studies have shown that even after thoracotomy with complete lung palpation, recurrence in the ipsilateral lung is as common or even more likely than in the contralateral lung, suggesting that even with bi-manual palpation small nodules may be missed [18,19].

More than 50% of patients are likely to have metastatic disease develop after resection of metastases. Re-resection has been shown to be an acceptable therapy and should be considered when patients present with recurrent pulmonary metastases [20]. Reoperative thoracotomies may be associated with significant adhesions from the previous operation. It could be argued that a VATS approach as the first procedure may minimize adhesion formation, possibly allowing a VATS approach on a second operation, which could be better-tolerated.

Probably the best data supporting the use of VATS come from a study examining the use of the technique in patients with colorectal metastases. Colorectal carcinoma is the second most common visceral malignancy in the United States, with an incidence of approximately 130,000 cases per year. Although the recurrence of disease is mainly locoregional, in 20%

of cases the recurrences are distant. The lungs are the most common site of extra-abdominal disease. It is estimated that isolated metastases to the lung occurs in 2% to 4% of all patients with colorectal cancer [21]. The largest multicenter series of VATS resections for metastatic colon cancer involved 80 patients [1] A solitary lesion was resected in 60 (75%) and multiple lesions in 20 (25%) patients. Only four (5%) patients required conversion to an open procedure. Mean survival was 30.4 months for patients with single tumors compared with 26.5 months for patients with multiple tumors. Sixty-nine percent (55/80) of the patients eventually had recurrence develop, with most (38% of the original 80 patients) having distant recurrences. The mean disease-free interval in those patients who have not had recurrence was 38.7 months. The authors concluded that VATS was efficacious but that conversion to thoracotomy should be performed if any of the lesions seen on CT are not identified, or if margins were inadequate.

Adjuncts to video-assisted thoracic surgery

If the metastasis is directly subpleural, a mound will often form on the surface of the lung as the surrounding lung becomes atelectatic, and the tumor will be easily identified. If the mass is deeper, it can often be identified by passing a blunt probe over the surface of the lung or by placing a finger through a port incision. In some cases, however, the mass will be too small and too deep to be identified by these methods. Similar to mammographic needle localization, placement of a guide wire by CT guidance into the lesion can be performed [22]. Methylene blue marking may also used either alone or in conjunction with needle localization to facilitate identification during VATS of the area to be resected, and it is particularly useful should the guide wire dislodge during transfer of the patient from CT to the operating room. One series of guide wire localization biopsies involved 101 localizations in 94 patients [22]. Six patients had more than one nodule localized. The wire dislodged from the lung in 22 cases; however, methylene blue staining allowed localization without extra ports or digital palpation. Overall, the nodule was within the first wedge biopsy of lung tissue in 98% of the resected specimens.

More recently, an approach using CT-guided placement of platinum microcoils has been described for small pulmonary nodules [23]. With this technique, the distal end of the coil is place adjacent to the nodule and the superficial end coiled at the pleural surface. This technique was found to be a 100%

effective in a phase I study involving 12 patients with pulmonary nodules.

Another technique that may help in identification of small nodules is that of hand-assisted thorascopic surgery (HATS). HATS involves VATS with the addition of a hand port to help identify smaller lesions that may be undectected by standard radiographic imaging. Wright and colleagues described the use of HATS in 46 patients with only two conversions to open operation [24]. With their technique, a 7- to 8-cm incision is made 2 cm below the costal margin and extended through the rectus muscle. The fingers are passed behind the costal margin staying in the extraperitoneal plane. The diaphragm is then split in the line of the anterior diaphragmatic fibers, near the periphery, to minimize injury to the phrenic nerve. It is then possible to place a hand to palpate the lung, localize the nodule, and better estimate margin during resection of a nodule. More recently, Detterbeck and his group used a handport during thoracoscopic resection of metastatic pulmonary disease in 24 consecutive patients [25]. They describe a different technique that involves a midline epigastric incision with an extraplueral dissection. The fascial attachments to the xiphoid are divided and the xiphoid is removed. They found that 67% of their cases were completed without conversion to an open procedure. The rate of incomplete resection and recurrence was comparable to that of open procedures.

Video-assisted thoracic surgery: patient selection

Suggested selection criteria for VATS metastectomy listed here are similar to those for open metastectomy.

- Primary neoplasm controlled or controllable
- Helical CT scan (thin cut)
- Limited number of metastases (2 or fewer)
- Ability to tolerate resection (based on lung function and cardiac evaluation)
- Tumor nodules in outer 1/3 of lung
- All thoracic metastatic disease resectable by VATS

If multiple probable sites of disease (defined as more than 2) are present, we recommend an open approach, because the likelihood of radiologically occult metastases is great. We acknowledge, however, that the clinical benefit of removing these occult metastases is unclear and that in some centers VATS resection may be performed only for patients with very limited disease. VATS is a good option as a

diagnostic tool for the indeterminate nodule, or in a patient with multiple nodules, for which a diagnosis is required before initiating medical therapies. Most surgeons accept VATS as a compromise operation for the patient at high risk for complications after a thoracotomy.

Radiofrequency ablation

Background

Radiofrequency ablation (RFA) is a relatively new ablative modality that is gaining popularity as therapy for lung tumors [26]. RFA is a thermal energy system that functions by delivering an alternating current that passes from active to dispersive and back to the active electrodes. This results in frictional and resistive heating. When normal cells are exposed to temperatures greater than 60°C, cells will die. Cancer cells, however, are inherently more sensitive to heat and can be killed by temperatures as low as 41°C [27]. RF ablation systems will typically heat local tissue to temperatures as high as 100°C, resulting in coagulative necrosis of tumors. An RFA system consists of three components: a generator, an active electrode that is placed within a tumor, and dispersive electrodes (electrosurgical return pads) that are placed on the patient.

RFA has been successfully used for treatment of primary and metastatic hepatic lesions, with necrosis rates of 70% to 98% [28]. Animal models have been used to investigate the efficacy and feasibility of this technique in lung tissue. In a study by Goldberg and colleagues, the authors generated a model of lung tumors by infiltrating the pulmonary parenchyma of 11 rabbits with VX2 sarcoma cell suspensions [29]. Seven lesions were treated with RFA for 6 minutes at 90°C, and the remaining four tumors were untreated as controls. The authors noted CT evidence of coagulation necrosis surrounding the tumor, manifested by increased opacity enveloping the lesion, followed by central tissue attenuation with peripheral hyper-attenuation surrounding the treated site. Histological analysis revealed that at least 95% of the tumor nodules were necrotic, although some rabbits (43%) had residual tumor nests at the periphery of the tumor. Pneumothorax was the only procedure-related complication, and this occurred in 29% of treated rabbits and in 25% of controls. In another study, Miao and colleagues implanted VX2 tumor tissue in the lung of 18 rabbits (12 treated and 6 controls), and the lesions were then treated with RFA using a cooled-tip electrode for 60 seconds [30]. Absolute tumor eradication with RFA was achieved in 33% of rabbits that survived more than 3 months. Microangiography revealed no perfusion to the ablated lesion. On histopathological evaluation, the ablated lesion retained its tissue architecture, but with changes consistent with coagulation necrosis with surrounding edema and inflammation of normal surrounding lung. After 1 to 3 months of treatment, the ablated tumor became an atrophied nodule of coagulation necrosis within a fibrotic capsule. The timing and progression of these postablation changes are an important issue when evaluating treatment response and are discussed later.

Clinical experience with radiofrequency ablation

Following the clinical experience with liver tumors and with animal models of lung malignancies, RFA has been used in clinical practice to treat lung tumors. The first published report was in 2000, and it demonstrated the feasibility of this technique in three patients with lung tumors [26]. Since then, a number of case reports and series have been published, with most demonstrating safety and feasibility of the technique [31,32].

We have been treating patients since 2000. In our initial reported experience, we treated 33 tumors in 18 patients [33]. Tumor pathologies included metastatic carcinoma (8), sarcoma (5), or lung cancer (5). Mean age was 60 years (range, 27 to 95). Initially, RFA was performed by mini-thoracotomy (n = 5) but as experience was gained with this modality, our preferred approach has been using CT-guided percutaneous ablation (n = 13) under general anesthesia. In the CT-guided procedures, a small finder needle is placed into the center of the lung nodule. After confirming successful placement with CT imaging, the active RFA electrode is then placed into the lesion and deployed (Fig. 1). The needle electrode size is chosen according to the diameter of the target lesion. Generally, we strive to achieve an ablation zone that is at least 1 cm larger than the nodule.

Chest tubes were required in 7 of 13 (53.8%) percutaneous procedures in this series. These were for small pneumothoraces that developed during the procedure and most were removed within 24 hours. Mean hospitalization was 3 days (range, 1 to 7 days). Complications included delayed pneumothorax (1/18), pneumonitis (4/18), small pleural effusion (9/18), and transient renal failure (1/18). One death occurred from massive hemoptysis 19 days after RFA of a central nodule. This patient had also received recent brachytherapy for an endobronchial tumor. As a result of this death, we do not recommend percutaneous RFA for central tumors. Treatment results were

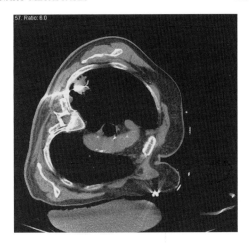

Fig. 1. CT image demonstrating deployed radiofrequency ablation probe in tumor.

better with smaller tumors. At a mean follow-up of 6 months (range, 1 to 14 months), CT revealed a radiographically determined response in 8 of 12 patients (66%) with tumors smaller than 5 cm, compared with two of six (33.3%) in patients with tumors larger than 5 cm. Similarly, 66% of patients with tumors 5 cm or larger died during the follow-up period, compared with 33% of patients with tumors 5 cm or less.

As a result of this study, we have limited the use of RFA to tumors 5 cm or less. We recently reported our experience with non-small cell lung cancer [34]. Median tumor diameter was 2.8 cm, and 50% of the patients had stage I disease. Local progression occurred in 38.1% of the nodules at a median progression-free interval of 18 months.

For pulmonary metastases, as with the open and VATS literature, the biggest reports for RFA are with treating metastatic colorectal cancer. Steinke and colleagues reported on 23 patients who had 52 metastases ablated [35]. Pneumothorax occurred in 43% of the patients. Five patients (21.7%) died of further metastatic disease. A malignant pleural effusion developed in one patient. Eighteen patients with 40 nodules had follow-up at 1 year. Among the 40 nodules, 17 (42.5%) had disappeared, 5 (12.5%) had decreased, 4 (10%) were stable, and 14 (35%) had increased in size.

A recent study combined results of RFA from seven centers around the world [36] providing primarily morbidity and mortality data on a total of 493 cases. The authors concluded that RFA was safe with negligible mortality, little morbidity, and a gain in quality of life. Although we agree that RFA

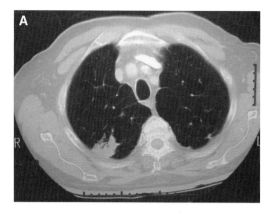 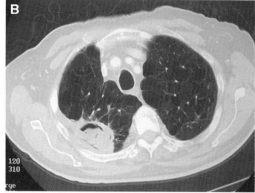

Fig. 2. (*A*) CT image demonstrating tumor before radiofrequency ablation. (*B*) CT image 3 months after radiofrequency ablation. Cavitation and bubble lucencies are demonstrated, as well as surrounding scar tissue.

is safe in comparison to pulmonary resection [37], the authors did not provide any data supporting their claim of improved quality of life. Is should also be emphasized that patients with limited metastatic disease or solitary pulmonary nodules are unlikely to be symptomatic and as such are unlikely to gain significant subjective benefit from treatment.

Outcome assessment

A challenging problem is the assessment of treatment response after RFA. Unlike an operation in which a cancer is removed, after RFA there is usually a significant residual mass, and determining whether there is residual or recurrent disease may be difficult. In the animal experiments discussed, we alluded to the observation of central necrosis that is usually surrounded by a rim of edema and in-flammation [30]. After approximately 3 months, the ablated area becomes an atrophied nodule of coagu-lation necrosis within a fibrotic capsule. Clinically,

the lesion often appears larger after ablation (Figs. 2A and 2B) and does not start to shrink for 3 months, when presumably the inflammatory changes have started to subside [38,39]. We have been using a modification of the RECIST criteria to assess ab-lated tumors at follow-up (Table 1). This combines elements of the size and quality of the ablated mass with PET information to make the determination of disease progression or regression in the ablated nodule. Other centers have been exploring the use of CT densitometry protocols to help evaluate for persistent or recurrent disease [40]. Densitometry is time-consuming and of value only to those patients with single nodules. Densitometry therefore would not be applicable to many patients with pulmonary metatstases. Beause the changes after RFA have often only started to subside by 3 months, the 3-month CT scan can be regarded as a baseline study [39]. Further growth in size or progressive FDG avidity on PET imaging after 3 months are likely to represent tumor progression. To study this further, the American

Table 1
Modified RECIST criteria used to evaluate treatment response

Response	CT mass size (recist)	CT mass quality	PET
Complete (Two of the following)	Lesion disappearance or scar <25% of original size	Cyst/cavity formation Low density of entire lesion	SUV <2.5
Partial (One of the following)	More than 30% decrease in the LD of target lesion	Central necrosis or central cavitation with liquid density	Decreased SUV or FDG uptake
Stable lesion (One of the following)	Less than 30% decrease in the LD of target lesion	Mass solid appearance, no central necrosis or cavity	Unchanged SUV or FDG uptake
Progression (Two of the following)	Increase of more than 20% in LD of target lesion	Solid mass, invasion adjacent structures	Higher SUV

Target lesions, tumors treated with RFA; LD, largest diameter of target (RFA treated) lesions; SUV, standard uptake value of 18-FDG in PET scan.

College of Surgeons Oncology Group (ACOSOG) will be opening a study later this year (ACOSOG Z4033) that will address the issue of local control after RFA for non-small cell lung cancer. The study will include serial CT scan (with densitometry) as well as PET scans. Hopefully, the information gained from this study will help define the optimal method of following patients after RFA.

Radiofrequency ablation: patient selection

The experience with RFA is still relatively small, with most series demonstrating only safety and feasibility. As mentioned, determination of local control is still challenging. Unlike resection (with either a VATS or open approach), margins are not available. Although we strive to ablate an area at least 1 cm greater than the largest diameter of the tumor, 100% ablation may not always be achieved. In one multicenter study of 15 patients, RFA was performed at thoracotomy immediately before resection of the tumor [41]. Ablation was possible in 13 cases. In these 13 patients median tumor kill was 70%, with seven patients achieving 100% ablation. There appeared to be a learning curve effect, with five of the last six cases achieving 100% ablation. This study demonstrates that RFA can produce effective ablation; however, in the absence of 100% guaranteed cell death in every case, resection should continue to be the favored approach for patients whenever possible.

Suggested selection criteria for RFA are outlined below.

- Primary neoplasm controlled or controllable
- Helical CT scan (thin cut)
- Limited number of metastases (3 or fewer)
- All tumor nodules 5cm or less
- Patient should be felt not to be a candidate for resection by thoracic surgeon
- Tumor nodules should be in the outer 2/3 of the lung (ie, should not abut mediastinum)
- All thoracic disease amenable to RFA

These are similar to those for VATS; however, RFA should be regarded as a compromise for the patient who is felt to be at increased risk for pulmonary resection. One exception to this may be the patient who presents with recurrent ipsilateral disease after a previous thoracotomy. The morbidity of redo-thoracotomy is higher than a first-time thoracotomy. Additionally, such a patient has at least a 60% chance of re-presenting with recurrent disease in the future, even after reoperative thoracotomy [19]. RFA provides a good minimally invasive alternative for at least local control and possibly for cure in such patients. In addition to allowing treatment of patients at high risk, RFA may allow surgeons to treat patients who may not meet traditional criteria for pulmonary metastectomy. For instance, we have used RFA to ablate colorectal metastases to the lung in patients who have also undergone RFA of liver metastases. Thoracotomy is not appropriate when these patients have already undergone a compromise procedure (instead of resection) for their liver metastases. Similarly, in patients with impaired pulmonary function, we have performed wedge resection of peripheral metastases and RFA for central lesions to avoid lobectomy.

Summary

Therapeutic pulmonary metastectomy is accepted therapy for pulmonary metastases. However, more than 50% of patients who undergo this treatment will experience recurrences, many within the same lobe. Minimally invasive approaches provide an option for therapy that minimizes morbidity and, in the case of RFA, preserves pulmonary function. The long-term results of RFA, even for non-small cell lung cancer, are not yet determined. Resection using a VATS or open approach should continue to remain the standard of care.

References

[1] Landreneau RJ, De Giacomo T, Mack MJ, et al. Therapeutic video-assisted thoracoscopic surgical resection of colorectal pulmonary metastases. Eur J Cardiothorac Surg 2000;18:671–6 [discussion 676–7].
[2] Long-term results of lung metastasectomy: prognostic analyses based on 5206 cases. The International Registry of Lung Metastases. J Thorac Cardiovasc Surg 1997;113:37–49.
[3] Pastorino U. Lung metastasectomy: why, when, how. Crit Rev Oncol Hematol 1997;26:137–45.
[4] Landreneau RJ, Mack MJ, Hazelrigg SR, et al. Prevalence of chronic pain after pulmonary resection by thoracotomy or video-assisted thoracic surgery. J Thorac Cardiovasc Surg 1994;107:1079–85 [discussion 1085–6].
[5] Dowling RD, Wachs ME, Ferson PF, et al. Thoracoscopic neodymium: yttrium aluminum garnet laser resection of a pulmonary metastasis. Cancer 1992;70:1873–5.

[6] Champion JK, Delisle N, Hunt T. Comparison of thoracoscopic and laproscopic esophagomyotomy with fundoplication for primary motility disorders. Eur J Cardiothorac Surg 1999;16(Suppl 1):S34–6.

[7] Demmy TL, James TA, Swanson SJ, et al. Trouble-shooting video-assisted thoracic surgery lobectomy. Ann Thorac Surg 2005;79:1744–52 [discussion 1753].

[8] Luketich JD, Alvelo-Rivera M, Buenaventura PO, et al. Minimally invasive esophagectomy: outcomes in 222 patients. Ann Surg 2003;238:486–94 [discussion 494–485].

[9] McCormack PM, Bains MS, Begg CB, et al. Role of video-assisted thoracic surgery in the treatment of pulmonary metastases: results of a prospective trial. Ann Thorac Surg 1996;62:213–6 [discussion 216–7].

[10] Girard P, Baldeyrou P, Le Chevalier T, et al. Surgery for pulmonary metastases. Who are the 10-year survivors? Cancer 1994;74:2791–7.

[11] Gadd MA, Casper ES, Woodruff JM, et al. Development and treatment of pulmonary metastases in adult patients with extremity soft tissue sarcoma. Ann Surg 1993;218:705–12.

[12] Mutsaerts EL, Zoetmulder FA, Meijer S, et al. Outcome of thoracoscopic pulmonary metastasectomy evaluated by confirmatory thoracotomy. Ann Thorac Surg 2001;72:230–3.

[13] Mutsaerts EL, Zoetmulder FA, Meijer S, et al. Long term survival of thoracoscopic metastasectomy vs metastasectomy by thoracotomy in patients with a solitary pulmonary lesion. Eur J Surg Oncol 2002;28:864–8.

[14] Margaritora S, Porziella V, D'Andrilli A, et al. Pulmonary metastases: can accurate radiological evaluation avoid thoracotomic approach? Eur J Cardiothorac Surg 2002;21:1111–4.

[15] Ninomiya M, Nakajima J, Tanaka M, et al. Effects of lung metastasectomy on respiratory function. Jpn J Thorac Cardiovasc Surg 2001;49:17–20.

[16] Landreneau RJ, Mack MJ, Keenan RJ, et al. Strategic planning for video-assisted thoracic surgery. Ann Thorac Surg 1993;56:615–9.

[17] Roth JA, Pass HI, Wesley MN, et al. Comparison of median sternotomy and thoracotomy for resection of pulmonary metastases in patients with adult soft-tissue sarcomas. Ann Thorac Surg 1986;42:134–8.

[18] Martini N, McCormack PM, Bains MS, et al. Surgery for solitary and multiple pulmonary metastases. N Y State J Med 1978;78:1711–4.

[19] Weiser MR, Downey RJ, Leung DH, et al. Repeat resection of pulmonary metastases in patients with soft-tissue sarcoma. J Am Coll Surg 2000;191:184–90 [discussion 190–1].

[20] Kandioler D, Kromer E, Tuchler H, et al. Long-term results after repeated surgical removal of pulmonary metastases. Ann Thorac Surg 1998;65:909–12.

[21] McCormack PM, Ginsberg RJ. Current management of colorectal metastases to lung. Chest Surg Clin North Am 1998;8:119–26.

[22] Thaete FL, Peterson MS, Plunkett MB, et al. Computed tomography-guided wire localization of pulmo-

nary lesions before thoracoscopic resection: results in 101 cases. J Thorac Imaging 1999;14:90–8.

[23] Powell TI, Jangra D, Clifton JC, et al. Peripheral lung nodules: fluoroscopically guided video-assisted thoracoscopic resection after computed tomography-guided localization using platinum microcoils. Ann Surg 2004;240:481–8 [discussion 488–9].

[24] Wright GM, Clarke CP, Paiva JM. Hand-assisted thoracoscopic surgery. Ann Thorac Surg 2003;75:1665–7.

[25] Detterbeck FC, Egan TM. Thoracoscopy using a substernal handport for palpation. Ann Thorac Surg 2004;78:1031–6.

[26] Dupuy DE, Zagoria RJ, Akerley W, et al. Percutaneous radiofrequency ablation of malignancies in the lung. AJR Am J Roentgenol 2000;174:57–9.

[27] Giovanella BC, Lohman WA, Heidelberger C. Effects of elevated temperatures and drugs on the viability of L1210 leukemia cells. Cancer Res 1970;30:1623–31.

[28] Curley SA, Izzo F. Laparoscopic radiofrequency. Ann Surg Oncol 2000;7:78–9.

[29] Goldberg SN, Gazelle GS, Compton CC, et al. Radiofrequency tissue ablation of VX2 tumor nodules in the rabbit lung. Acad Radiol 1996;3:929–35.

[30] Miao Y, Ni Y, Bosmans H, et al. Radiofrequency ablation for eradication of pulmonary tumor in rabbits. J Surg Res 2001;99:265–71.

[31] Schaefer O, Lohrmann C, Langer M. CT-guided radiofrequency ablation of a bronchogenic carcinoma. Br J Radiol 2003;76:268–70.

[32] VanSonnenberg E, Shankar S, Morrison PR, et al. Radiofrequency ablation of thoracic lesions: part 2, initial clinical experience–technical and multidisciplinary considerations in 30 patients. AJR Am J Roentgenol 2005;184:381–90.

[33] Herrera LJ, Fernando HC, Perry Y, et al. Radiofrequency ablation of pulmonary malignant tumors in nonsurgical candidates. J Thorac Cardiovasc Surg 2003;125:929–37.

[34] Fernando HC, De Hoyos A, Landreneau RJ, et al. Radiofrequency ablation for the treatment of non-small cell lung cancer in marginal surgical candidates. J Thorac Cardiovasc Surg 2005;129:639–44.

[35] Steinke K, Glenn D, King J, et al. Percutaneous imaging-guided radiofrequency ablation in patients with colorectal pulmonary metastases: 1-year follow-up. Ann Surg Oncol 2004;11:207–12.

[36] Steinke K, Sewell PE, Dupuy D, et al. Pulmonary radiofrequency ablation–an international study survey. Anticancer Res 2004;24:339–43.

[37] Ginsberg RJ, Hill LD, Eagan RT, et al. Modern thirty-day operative mortality for surgical resections in lung cancer. J Thorac Cardiovasc Surg 1983;86:654–8.

[38] Steinke K, King J, Glenn D, et al. Radiologic appearance and complications of percutaneous computed tomography-guided radiofrequency-ablated pulmonary metastases from colorectal carcinoma. J Comput Assist Tomogr 2003;27:750–7.

[39] Bojarski JD, Dupuy DE, Mayo-Smith WW. CT Imaging Findings of Pulmonary Neoplasms After Treatment with Radiofrequency Ablation: Results in 32 Tumors. AJR Am J Roentgenol 2005;185: 466–71.

[40] Suh RD, Wallace AB, Sheehan RE, et al. Unresectable pulmonary malignancies: CT-guided percutaneous radiofrequency ablation–preliminary results. Radiology 2003;229:821–9.

[41] Yang SWR, Askin F, Whyte R, et al. Radiofrequency ablation of primary and metastatic lung tumors; Analysis of an ablate and resect study. Paper presented at: American Association for Thoracic Surgery 82nd Annual Meeting, 2002; Washington, DC.

THORACIC
SURGERY
CLINICS

Thorac Surg Clin 16 (2006) 167 – 183

Pulmonary Metastasectomy in Pediatric Patients

Mark L. Kayton, MD

*Division of Pediatric Surgery, Department of Surgery, Memorial Sloan-Kettering Cancer Center, 1275 York Avenue,
New York, NY 10021, USA*

It is now generally accepted that infants and children can readily withstand thoracotomy, that some children who have cancer and lung metastases can achieve long-term survival and even cure following metastasectomy, and that nonanatomic wedge resection is an ideal technique to perform metastasectomy while preserving lung parenchyma. These observations, however, are the culmination of 50 years of retrospective study in the pediatric population. To reach these broad conclusions, pediatric surgeons frequently compiled case series that, out of necessity, grouped together patients who had broadly dispersed histologies. Together, this body of literature establishes that pediatric pulmonary metastasectomy can be performed safely, but the question of whether metastasectomy should be performed on a particular patient has only recently come into focus. The indications for metastasectomy in pediatric patients vary greatly and are sometimes diametrically opposed depending on the primary tumor type.

Historical background

Pulmonary metastasectomy for solid tumors in children began to enter into practice in the 1950s and the literature in the early 1960s. In what may colloquially be referred to as one of the first pediatric multi-institutional studies, Richardson [1] in 1961 reported the results of a written survey of pediatric and thoracic surgeons in which an accumulated experience with 35 children undergoing pulmonary

metastasectomy yielded 8 patients who were 5-year survivors. White and Krivit [2] reported in 1962 on the 10-year survival of a boy who had two metastatic deposits of Wilms tumor removed from his lung and on an apparent cure (with 5 years' follow-up) of a boy with rhabdosarcoma metastatic to the lung. Although one may reasonably expect the literature to be enriched with more favorable reports than with disastrous ones, the stage was nonetheless set for optimism for the pursuit of pulmonary metastasectomy in children.

By 1967, several large case series were published. Cliffton and Pool [3] wrote of their experience with 27 pediatric metastasectomies between 1952 and 1967. These investigators made the following points:

1. Multiplicity of metastases should not be a contraindication to operation.
2. The type of tumor is important.
3. A short time-to-development of metastases should not prohibit consideration of resection of the metastases.
4. Staged, bilateral resections are well tolerated.
5. Diagnostic uncertainty can be addressed well by thoracotomy and may save a child the toxicity from un-needed adjuvant therapy if the pathology proves benign.

Although their series lumped together patients who had numerous different histologies, the points that these investigators were able to distill are of lasting value to us today.

The technique of wedge resection (although continued to be debated for many years [4]) was argued to be a safe alternative to segmental resection or lobectomy in a remarkable compilation of 55 children

E-mail address: kaytonm@mskcc.org

reported by Kilman and colleagues [5] in 1969. Of the 84 total resections performed in these patients, 40 or almost half were wedge resections, many with good results. A 36% 5-year survival rate was found. The investigators wrote that "bilateral lesions, multiple lesions, or lesions present at time of resection of the primary tumor, should not contraindicate surgical resection of the pulmonary metastases."

In 1971, a huge advance in the importance of pulmonary metastasectomy in children occurred when Martini and colleagues [6] at Memorial Sloan-Kettering Cancer Center wrote of their results in patients who had osteosarcoma. Without resection, pulmonary metastases from osteosarcoma had historically been associated with a grim 5% survival at 3 years from diagnosis [7]. After undergoing metastasectomy, however, 9 of 20 osteosarcoma patients (45%) were alive 3 years from diagnosis. As many as seven thoracotomies per patient were required. Several of these patients went on to become long-term (>20-year) survivors [8].

By the early 1970s, therefore, the physiologic tolerance of most children to thoracotomy for metastasectomy was no longer in question. It had additionally been established that some children could achieve long-term survival and even cure, and moreover, that this result could often be accomplished by wedge resection. What followed over the next 3 decades was a disappointing lull in progress in understanding the indications for pediatric metastasectomy. Faced with small numbers of patients who had any particular disease at a given medical center, surgeons tended to group together patients of vastly disparate histologies when writing reviews and case series. In the series from Kilman and colleagues [5], the histologies included Wilms tumor, osteosarcoma, rhabdomyosarcoma, neuroblastoma, and no fewer than eight other types of tumor metastatic to the lungs. Barrows and Kmetz [9], who in 1975 reported that six of seven pediatric lobectomy patients were long-term cancer survivors, included children in their series who had Wilms tumor, osteosarcoma, and soft tissue sarcoma.

Astonishingly, case series right up to the present time continue to be hampered by this problem. In a 2004 report on metastasectomy in 44 pediatric patients, Torre and colleagues [10] again conglomerated Wilms tumor patients with children who had sarcomas and germ cell tumors. Because of this attempt to analyze multiple different entities together, the investigators were unable to make any determinations except that the overall 5-year survival rate was 53.8%. They regrettably concluded that metastasectomy "remains an open question" and that "there is a role

for surgery, but only if this is performed as part of a multi-disciplinary concept of treatment...." This statement could well have been made 30 years earlier and, in fact, it had been [9].

The proper application of pulmonary metastasectomy to children revolves around the particular histology being treated. This was plainly stated by Heij and colleagues [11] in 1994 who wrote, "the most important prognostic factor is the type of primary tumor." For some tumors (eg, adrenocortical carcinoma), the absence of any significant responses to chemotherapy and radiotherapy promote metastasectomy to a much more central role. For other tumors such as osteosarcoma, a large series has now validated the use of aggressive resection of all clinically detectable disease. For neuroblastoma and several other tumor types discussed in this article, the application of pulmonary metastasectomy must be tailored to each individual case. Many pediatric cancers are susceptible to chemotherapy and to radiation-based or nuclear medicine–based therapies, and the relative toxicities of these alternative therapies factor into any decision about metastasectomy.

In this article, the author considers common pitfalls in the diagnosis of pulmonary metastases in pediatric patients, discusses specialized techniques for the biopsy of pulmonary lesions in children, summarizes the indications for metastasectomy in the tumors commonly encountered in young patients, and describes technical issues related to the performance of thoracotomy in pediatric surgery.

Pitfalls in diagnostic techniques

Since the 1979 prospective study from Chang and colleagues [12] at the National Cancer Institute showing that CT scanning was more sensitive than conventional tomography for the detection of small pulmonary nodules in patients who had metastatic disease, CT has been a trusted modality for the detection of pulmonary metastases, as much so in children as in adults. Two noteworthy exceptions exist in pediatric cancer, however. Wilms tumor staging has classically relied on conventional chest radiographs [13]. It has been difficult to demonstrate that patients who have "CT-only" lung nodules fare more poorly in a statistically significant way [14–16]. Another exception is in pediatric thyroid cancer, whereby the radiotracer uptake of ^{131}I in pulmonary micrometastases may occur despite a normal chest radiograph [17] and, therefore, may prompt treatment for metastatic disease in the lungs.

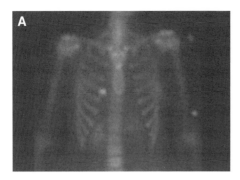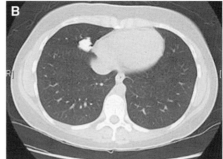

Fig. 1. (*A*) Technitium 99m bone scan image showing uptake in a particularly large pulmonary metastasis of osteosarcoma. (*B*) CT image of the same lesion.

Other modalities have shown inconsistent reliability in the detection of pediatric pulmonary metastases. Bone scanning can at times be extraordinary in highlighting large lung metastases from osteosarcoma but is not the recommended modality for detecting lung metastases because it requires that the lesions be sizable and active (Fig. 1). Thoracoscopic ultrasound has recently been described for the localization of pediatric lung lesions (Gow et al, submitted for publication, 2006), but the validation of this technique for the detection of individual malignant histologies, which vary in density depending on the diagnosis, has yet to be performed.

Although often prompting calls for surgical consultation, abnormal findings on pediatric chest CT scans must be considered critically within their clinical context. Ill children, especially those requiring anesthesia for bone marrow aspiration, for lumbar punctures, or even for the performance of the CT scan itself, are prone to exhibiting atelectasis that may be

mistaken for malignancy in the lung (Fig. 2). Attention to the technique and clinical context of the scan is therefore paramount, and repetition of the scan may be warranted if uncertainty exists.

Even when a lesion proves nonartifactual, it is difficult to distinguish benign from malignant processes on pediatric CT scans. This difficulty has been verified in a number of studies in which pediatric radiologists have evaluated, in blinded fashion, their own readings in comparison with postoperative pathologic diagnoses. Rosenfield and colleagues [18] found that in the case of tiny nodules on pediatric CT scans, an accurate diagnosis of benign versus malignant could not be rendered preoperatively when validated against the pathology results obtained at open biopsy. McCarville and colleagues [19], in a study of the CT diagnosis of osteosarcoma metastases, found that calcification in a lesion was not a reliable indicator of the malignancy of the lesion.

Thus, the surgeon must often assume the risk of thoracic exploration or biopsy on the basis of limited predictive information. To this end, the surgeon should take into account the potential benefits that can stem from providing a tissue diagnosis for patients and their families (who will often gladly undergo even a thoracotomy to achieve certainty that a nodule is not malignant) and for oncologists and radiation oncologists (whose treatment plans may be affected substantially). Initial inclinations to have suspicious nodules examined by biopsy using noninvasive means, rather than proceeding with exploration of the chest, are not always the best course either: for some disease processes, the patient's survival depends on the complete detection and resection of all deposits of metastatic disease. An illustration of this predicament is depicted in Fig. 3, which shows the chest CT scans of four patients who had osteosarcoma. All underwent complete, open exploration of the involved hemithorax at the author's institution on

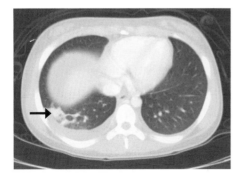

Fig. 2. Atelectasis at the base of the right lung (*arrow*) in a patient who had rhabdomyosarcoma and a pleural effusion. This patient had undergone sedation earlier the same day for bone marrow biopsy. On the basis of the CT scan, one cannot reliably distinguish atelectasis from metastasis.

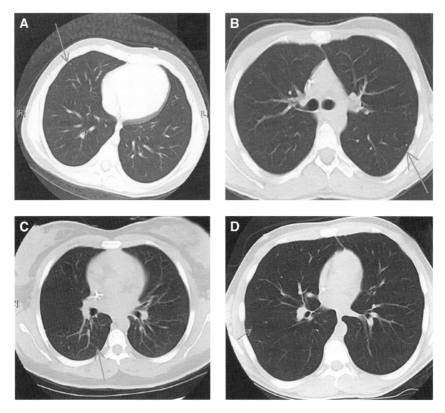

Fig. 3. CT scans depicting lung lesions (*arrows*) in four patients who had osteosarcoma. Pathologically, the lesion in (*A*) proved to be interstitial fibrosis with foreign body giant cell reaction; the lesion in (*B*) was a benign calcification; the lesion in (*C*) represented metastatic osteosarcoma; and the lesion in (*D*) corresponded to a benign intraparenchymal lymph node.

the basis of suspicious CT scans. All had previously received chemotherapy. In three of these patients, the lung nodules proved benign, but the fourth patient was found to have (in addition to the lesion depicted in the figure) five other lesions that were not seen on CT. All six lesions were metastatic osteosarcoma. Because the other five lesions were not localized on CT and not pleural based, alternative biopsy techniques and even thoracoscopy would have been impossible strategies to employ. (Answers as to the pathologic diagnosis of the lesions in each of the four patients are found in the figure legend.)

Minimally invasive biopsy techniques for children

For situations that require biopsy alone, the application of minimally invasive techniques requires coordination among the appropriate radiologic, anesthetic, and surgical teams. As a result, biopsies can be performed even on deep parenchymal lesions in children. Five reports in the recent pediatric literature detail specialized techniques.

Needle localization was performed for lung lesions in two pediatric patients at St. Jude, followed by thoracoscopic resection of the lesions [20]. The investigators described CT-guided deployment of a 20-gauge Kopans needle. At thoracoscopy, the lung was collapsed, leaving the involved area of lung tented-up to the pleural surface by the indwelling hooked needle. This technique allowed resection of lesions that were deep to the pleural surface, or thoracoscopically invisible, and was successful even in a patient as young as 1 year. A disadvantage was the need for the needle to remain in the right place from the time of localization, throughout the period of transport, to the time of thoracoscopy. Waldhausen and colleagues [21] described a technique to achieve higher certainty of resecting the right area by injecting 0.1 mL of methylene blue subpleurally in addition to leaving a Homer mammographic needle in place. Biopsies were performed successfully in three children despite the dislodgement of the needle (presumably because of coughing) in one of them.

Three other described techniques circumvent the requirement for an indwelling needle by means of staining the lung tissue. Partrick and colleagues [22] reported the preoperative localization of lung nodules in 12 children using CT-guided injection of 0.2 to 0.5 mL of methylene blue dye, following which the needle was withdrawn and the children taken directly to thoracoscopy. Diffusion of dye was not a problem, but one child had a nondiagnostic biopsy and underwent a repeat procedure.

Scorpio and colleagues [23], in a case report, described the co-injection of a drop of dilute barium along with the methylene blue in the vicinity of the lung nodule. This technique enabled intraoperative use of fluoroscopy for targeting and for confirmation (by radiography of the specimen) that the area of interest was indeed resected. A substantial series of 19 procedures by McConnell and colleagues [24] reviewed the CT-guided injection of 0.3 mL of methylene blue mixed with 3 mL of autologous blood, which resulted in diagnostic biopsies in every case performed and no problems with tissue diffusion.

The following sections consider indications for surgical metastasectomy in different pediatric tumor types.

Wilms tumor

Table 1 summarizes major series of pediatric metastasectomy for Wilms tumor, encompassing a 43-year period [1,3–5,11,25–33]. Other adjuvant therapies obviously varied greatly during this time span, and the case series were observational, retrospective series. Before the late 1980s, it can be seen that survival hovered around 50%, with reasonably long-term follow-up in many of the series. From 1988 onward, multiple factors (many of them nonsurgical) contributed to the observed improvement in survival.

Chemotherapy and whole-lung irradiation have long been established to produce responses in Wilms tumor with pulmonary metastases [34]; however, whole-lung irradiation, in particular, is associated with a subsequent 12% rate of diffuse interstitial pneumonitis [35]. A schism in the treatment of radiographically discovered pulmonary metastases from Wilms tumor has arisen, with North American centers employing radiation as a central modality and major European centers favoring surgical metastasectomy.

Implying that four deaths (5% of the Wilms tumor cases in the series) from interstitial pneumonitis were related to radiotherapy, Baldeyrou and coworkers [27], writing from Paris in 1984, advocated avoiding whole-lung irradiation in children who could undergo a satisfactory complete debulking of pulmonary metastases. Using the strategy of preoperative chemotherapy followed by pulmonary metastasectomy for stage IV patients, with radiation withheld except for isolated cases of inoperable metastases, several European centers in the 1980s demonstrated

Table 1
Survival after pulmonary metastasectomy for Wilms tumor

Reference	n	Survivors	Duration of follow-up
Richardson, 1961 [1]	17	4/17 (24%)	5 y
Cliffton and Pool, 1967 [3]	10	4/10 (40%)	Median, 12 mo
Kilman et al, 1969 [5]	8	6/8 (75%)	Median, 17.5 mo
Ballantine et al, 1975 [4]	6	3/6 (50%)	Median, 8 mo
Rodgers et al, 1980 [25]	5	0/5 (0%)	Not stated
Frenckner et al, 1982 [26]	9	3/9 (33%)	36–120 mo for 3 survivors
Baldeyrou et al, 1984 [27]	75	37/75 (50%)	48–180 mo
Lembke, 1986 [28]	7	4/7 (57%)	10–110 mo
Di Lorenzo and Collin, 1988 [29]	5	4/5 (80%)	Mean, 100 mo
de Kraker et al, 1990 [30]	36	30/36 (83%)	Mean, 48 mo
Heij et al, 1994 [11]	24	12/24 (50%)	6–220 mo
Green et al and NWTS-1, 2, 3, 1991 [31]			
Favorable histology, solitary lesion	13	77%	4 y
Favorable histology, multiple lesions	4	75%	4 y
Unfavorable histology, solitary lesion	4	25%	4 y
Unfavorable histology, multiple lesions	1	100%	4 y
Karnak et al, 2002 [32]	4	4/4 (100%)	Median, 33 mo
Abel et al, 2004 [33]	5	5/5 (100%)	Median, 76 mo

The number of patients with Wilms tumor is listed under "n," but many series discussed additional patients of other histologies that have been excluded for the purpose of this table. Nonsurgical therapies such as chemotherapy and whole-lung irradiation varied from series to series.
Abbreviation: NWTS, National Wilms' Tumor Studies.

5-year recurrence-free and actuarial survival rates of 83% [30].

Similarly optimistic survival statistics emerged from the North American cooperative group trials known as the National Wilms Tumor Studies (NWTS), but these good survival statistics have been achieved with pulmonary metastasectomy being relegated to a peripheral or absent role. The NWTS studies have assessed patients separately depending on whether they had favorable or unfavorable histology.

Data for favorable histology patients are available from NWTS-4, in which 172 stage IV, favorable-histology patients had an overall survival rate of 71.4% to 90.6%. The exact figure varied according to the particular chemotherapy regimen used and whether pulmonary metastases were visible on chest radiograph or only by CT. Surgical metastasectomy had little contribution to these results, being reserved only for some of the patients whose pulmonary nodules persisted for 2 weeks after chemotherapy and the delivery of 12 Gy of whole-lung radiation. Thirteen (7.6%) of the 172 stage IV patients developed interstitial pneumonitis following pulmonary irradiation, which the study group believed was an "infrequent" complication of radiotherapy. Thus, excellent survival has been accomplished with acceptable toxicity, but no defined role for metastasectomy, in this group [36].

The question of whether pulmonary metastasectomy benefits favorable-histology patients of lower stages who go on to subsequently relapse in the lungs was evaluated in 211 patients on NWTS-1, -2, and -3, the results of which were published by Green and colleagues [31] in 1991. Chemotherapy plus radiotherapy was compared with chemotherapy, radiotherapy, plus metastasectomy. For favorable-histology patients whose relapse was limited to a solitary pulmonary metastasis and whose therapy (surgical or chemotherapeutic) was instituted within 30 days of relapse, there was no added benefit to metastasectomy in the 4-year postrelapse survival. For favorable histology patients with multiple metastases, as well as for unfavorable histology patients with any number of metastases, there were not enough patients undergoing metastasectomy to make a proper statistical comparison.

With respect to patients who had diffuse anaplasia, only 14 patients who were stage IV at diagnosis were studied in NWTS-3 and -4 combined [37]. Metastasectomy was not reported in the context of pulmonary metastases from anaplastic Wilms tumor, so no conclusions can be drawn from this small group; however, given the bleak survival rate of stage IV patients reported in these studies (0%–16.7% at

4 years), there may be a role for further investigation of metastasectomy in these patients and in others who have refractory or recurrent Wilms tumor. At Memorial Sloan-Kettering Cancer Center, for example, surgeons have performed metastasectomies to render patients free of clinically detectable disease in preparation for planned bone marrow transplant.

In summary, favorable-histology Wilms tumor patients who have lung metastases exhibit excellent survival following chemotherapy and pulmonary irradiation, with acceptable rates of interstitial pneumonitis. At most American centers, aggressive surgical metastasectomy has failed to find a place in the standard treatment regimen of Wilms tumor metastatic to the lungs; however, biopsy of pulmonary nodules has an important role in saving patients from the toxicity of potentially unnecessary adjuvant treatments.

Neuroblastoma

Descriptions of pulmonary metastasectomy for neuroblastoma cannot readily be found due to the rarity with which neuroblastoma metastasizes to the pulmonary parenchyma, with an incidence at diagnosis of 0.4% to 3.2% and an incidence at first progression of 6.3% [38,39]. Patients older than 1 year who have MYCN amplification, which is a poor prognostic indicator in general, have higher odds of presenting with lung metastases than those who do not have MYCN amplification [39]. Death from disease has been the most common outcome when lung metastases are present. Concurrent metastases to other sites are usually present [40], so in most cases, systemic treatment options are more appropriate than metastasectomy. If the lungs appear to be the sole site of disease, however, surgical biopsy should be undertaken; one case report details how systemic therapy was withheld with disastrous outcome secondary to failure to obtain a tissue diagnosis on isolated pulmonary nodules [41].

Lung metastases from neuroblastoma may be pleural based, parenchymal, or both, as shown in Fig. 4.

Adrenocortical carcinoma in children

Unlike neuroblastoma, adrenocortical carcinoma frequently spreads to the lungs. A Memorial Sloan-Kettering Cancer Center series found that 45% of 33 adults who had stage IV disease had pulmonary metastases [42]. Clinical experience suggests that pediatric patients who have this disease share this

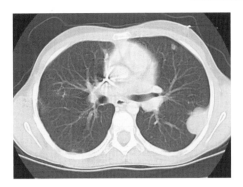

Fig. 4. Pulmonary metastases from neuroblastoma showing coexistence of pleural-based and parenchymal lesions in the left lung.

unfortunate tendency. Surgical metastasectomy is paramount in attempting to secure long-term survival in adrenocortical carcinoma. Although pediatric series of pulmonary metastasectomy for this disease do not exist, one should take to heart the adult data showing that resection of locally recurrent or distant metastatic disease is associated with a 57% 5-year survival rate, whereas incomplete resection of recurrences or metastases carries a 0% 5-year survival rate ($P<0.001$) [43]. For pulmonary metastases specifically, Memorial Sloan-Kettering Cancer Center data show a 71% 5-year survival rate for adults undergoing metastasectomy versus a 0% 5-year survival rate for those not undergoing metastasectomy [44]. Others similarly have found enhancement of survival in patients undergoing surgery for recurrences and metastases [45]. Common to all these reports, given the rarity of this disease, is the retrospective, non-randomized nature of the data. Thus, it may be the case that patients who had less aggressive or more unifocal disease were also the ones selected to undergo surgery.

Pediatric case reports, though, have clearly shown instances in which metastasectomy has been associated with long-term survival. An infant, reported by De León and colleagues [46] in 2002, underwent right lower lobectomy at age 8 months for metastatic adrenocortical carcinoma that had progressed on mitotane. The patient remained free of disease, with 15 years of follow-up reported. Appelqvist and Kostiainen [47] reported on a patient who underwent four thoracotomies for wedge resections of a total of nine pulmonary nodules after having had a adrenocortical primary excised at age 18 years; the patient was disease-free at 28 years of follow-up.

Metastasectomy for adrenocortical carcinoma should be performed early and should be complete.

Particular care should be taken to avoid tumor spillage. In the author's experience of four thoracotomies for this disease, metastases have been well encapsulated but gelatinous. Others have reported primary site spillage in 20% to 43% of operations for pediatric adrenocortical carcinoma [48]. The stakes of spillage are raised by the lack of any chemotherapy that can reliably prolong survival. Although ineffective, mitotane is used by many oncologists to treat adrenocortical carcinoma, and it must be remembered that lasting insufficiency of the remaining contralateral adrenal cortex may result from its use. In preparation for thoracotomy, stress steroids must be considered for patients treated with mitotane.

In contrast to those seen among adults, 90% of adrenocortical carcinomas in children are functional [49]. In these cases, recurrence of disease in the lungs may be determined by following secreted tumor markers. Urinary 17-ketosteroids are elevated in most children who have adrenocortical tumors [50]. Serum markers for recurrence should be sought for each patient on an individualized basis because functional tumors may differ in their predominant hormone production. The patient's initial clinical presentation may guide the surgeon and the endocrinologist as to whether the predominant hormone present is virilizing or feminizing or whether the patient has features of hyperaldosteronism or Cushing's syndrome. After they are determined, hormone markers should be measured before and after metastasectomy and followed at regular intervals thereafter. For example, the author found that serum androstenedione, dehydroepiandrosterone, and dehydroepiandrosterone sulfate were elevated in a 4-year-old who had an androgen-secreting metastatic adrenocortical carcinoma. These markers were subsequently useful for following recurrence. Imaging by CT remains important, but the author has not found positron emission tomography scanning to be helpful in this disease.

Osteosarcoma

There is probably no pediatric histology other than osteosarcoma for which metastasectomy is so clearly indicated. The data in the literature lend support to four concepts: (1) complete resection of osteosarcoma is associated with a survival benefit; (2) even when a chemotherapy "effect" is observed, surgical resection is still warranted; (3) preoperative radiologic findings are not predictive of the extent of disease that will be found intraoperatively; and (4) exploration of the contralateral lung is indicated in selected patients.

Before 1970, no patients who had pulmonary metastases from osteosarcoma survived beyond 5 years [7]. Since that time, multiagent chemotherapy and pulmonary metastasectomy have made important inroads in this disease. Case reports of dramatically long survival following pulmonary metastasectomy may now be found, such as the report by Hankins and DeSanto [50] showing the 25-year survival (and apparent cure) of a patient after right upper lobectomy for metastatic osteosarcoma. It is not merely resection but complete resection that is associated with a survival benefit; this has been shown in series by Schaller and colleagues [51] in 1982 and by Goorin and coworkers [52] in 1984.

More recently, large studies containing statistically meaningful survival analyses have emerged, which is a feature that cannot be claimed for most of the metastatic tumor types discussed in this article. In particular, Meyers and colleagues [53] showed in a group of 62 patients presenting with synchronous pulmonary metastases that complete resection of the primary tumor and all sites of metastatic disease was strongly correlated with overall survival ($P<0.001$); all 35 patients undergoing incomplete resection of all sites of measurable disease died. The German-Austrian-Swiss Osteosarcoma Study Group in 2003 analyzed 202 patients who presented with metastases at diagnosis and found that the completeness of surgical resection had a significant ($P=0.003$) impact on survival in multivariate analysis [54]. Resectability maintains a favorable impact on survival, even in the setting of second and third thoracotomies [55].

These data show that metastasectomy has a pivotal role in the treatment of metastatic osteosarcoma. Although chemotherapy is also indispensible in the treatment of osteosarcoma, it alone is not sufficient. Jaffe and colleagues [56] at M.D. Anderson Cancer Center performed a study in which primary osteosarcomas were left in situ when a pathologic response of complete necrosis could be ascertained on biopsy following chemotherapy. Even with the biopsy observation of "total tumor necrosis and fibrovascular regeneration," patients who had these lesions went on to develop local recurrences, metastases, and in most cases, death. Thus, complete excision is still advised, even when a lesion is thought likely to be necrotic after chemotherapy, a finding that should apply to metastases as rigorously as to the primary tumor.

A surgical technique must therefore be chosen to ensure that as complete a metastasectomy as possible is performed. At Memorial Sloan-Kettering Cancer Center, surgeons employ open thoracotomy to perform manual palpation of the entire lung for all patients explored for osteosarcoma. In a study of 54 thoracotomies for osteosarcoma, Kayton and colleagues [57] showed that the preoperative CT scan was an unreliable predictor of the number of metastases found intraoperatively, with a correlation coefficient of 0.45 ($P<0.001$). About half (47%) of the lesions were 5 mm or deeper from the pleural surface. Thoracoscopic surgery, which can only be used to resect lesions that have been identified on the preoperative scan or that are present on the pleural surface of the lung, is therefore not advised for complete metastasectomy in osteosarcoma.

Because the author and colleagues at Memorial Sloan-Kettering Cancer Center employ staged, bilateral thoracotomies whenever pulmonary metastasis is suspected, they are often faced with the decision as to whether to proceed with the second side. When a patient has resectable, histologically proved unilateral metastases from osteosarcoma and when the metastases occurs "early" in the disease (ie, within 2 years of initial diagnosis), Su and colleagues [58] showed that 78% of the time, metastases are found at exploration of the contralateral lung despite a negative CT scan on the contralateral side. Thus, the author and colleagues at Memorial Sloan-Kettering Cancer Center routinely perform staged, contralateral thoracotomy when patients meet these criteria. If the findings at the first thoracotomy are benign, then they do not proceed.

Nonrhabdomyosarcoma soft tissue sarcomas

Synovial cell sarcoma, chondrosarcoma, fibrosarcoma, and malignant fibrous histiocytoma are other pediatric sarcomatous tumors that may metastasize to the lung [59–61]. Owing to their rarity, they have not been studied nearly as well as osteosarcoma. Pulmonary metastases have not been observed to respond as favorably to whole-lung irradiation as they do in the case of, for instance, Ewing's sarcoma (see later discussion). Metastasectomy is advised as part of the multimodal therapy of these diseases [61,62]. The author approaches pulmonary metastases of these tumors with similar strategies as for osteosarcoma, although in the absence of osteoid matrix, the lesions in these diseases may be softer and more difficult to effectively palpate at thoracotomy.

Alveolar soft part sarcoma

This rare soft tissue sarcoma of young patients merits mention because of its predilection for metastasis to the lungs (Fig. 5). Alveolar soft part sarcoma

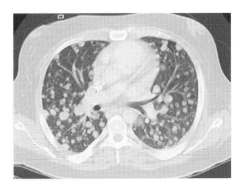

Fig. 5. Alveolar soft part sarcoma may be widely metastatic to the lungs.

strikes children and young adults, with a median age of diagnosis in the 20s [63,64]. Three pediatric case series have examined the course of the disease in younger patients. In the aggreggate 40 patients examined, there were only two partial responses to chemotherapy [65–67]; therefore, out of necessity, pulmonary metastasectomy figures centrally in the treatment of patients who have metastatic spread to the lungs unless insurmountable miliary involvement is already present.

Of 20 pediatric patients treated at Memorial Sloan-Kettering Cancer Center, 60% had lung metastases at presentation or subsequently [67]. Nine of the 20 patients had surgery for metastases, among them 17 thoracotomies and 2 thoracoscopies. One patient underwent 8 thoracotomies and was free of disease at last follow-up, 20 years following initial diagnosis. Alveolar soft part sarcoma grows indolently. Despite the presence of disease progression (the median 5-year progression-free survival rate was 22%), the author and colleagues observed a 5-year overall survival rate of 83% among pediatric patients. It cannot be determined whether the slow pace of the disease or the liberal application of metastasectomy accounts for this excellent overall survival in the face of progression of a disease for which there is no reliable role for chemotherapy or radiotherapy. Given the available data, however, pulmonary metastasectomy must continue to play a prominent role in the treatment of disseminated alveolar soft part sarcoma, and lifelong follow-up of these patients can help to diagnose progression before the extent of disease becomes surgically insurmountable.

Rhabdomyosarcoma

Results of pulmonary metastasectomy classically have been disappointing for this disease. Temeck and

colleagues [68] found that with respect to patients of other histologies, the 6 patients who had rhabdomyosarcoma undergoing thoracotomy in a retrospective study of 152 patients had a relative risk of 34.47 ($P<0.0001$, 95% confidence interval: 7.77–152.87) of having a shortened pulmonary progression-free interval. A 2004 report on metastasectomies for various histologies by Abel and coworkers [33] found that 3 of 3 patients who had rhabdomyosarcoma subjected to metastasectomy died within 36 months, 2 of them from cranial metastases.

Data from 46 patients who had isolated pulmonary metastases on the Intergroup Rhabdomyosarcoma Studies IV were analyzed by Rodeberg and colleagues [69] in 2005. Compared with children who had other sites of metastases, patients who had lung-only metastases were more likely to have favorable histology (embryonal, spindle cell, and botryoid), more likely to have parameningeal primaries rather than extremity primaries, and less likely to have nodal involvement. Only one fourth of these children underwent surgical confirmation of the lung disease by biopsy. Median survival was 2.15 years, and 79% of the children died of progression of disease. The major variable associated with prolonged failure-free and overall survival on multivariate analysis of the patients who had lung-only metastases was age less than 10 years. Administration of pulmonary radiotherapy appeared to provide benefits in failure-free and overall survival, although this was evaluated retrospectively and not randomized.

Given these data, the role of the surgeon for pulmonary metastatic disease in rhabdomyosarcoma should probably be limited to biopsy and to removal of isolated, stable metastases.

Ewing's sarcoma

Ewing's sarcomas are sensitive to chemotherapy and radiation [70], and the role of surgical metastasectomy has been variously reported across the spectrum from beneficial in selected patients [71] to "not warranted" [11]. Data from multiple case series of pediatric metastasectomy are condensed in Table 2 [1,4,11,25–29,32,68,71–75]. One may reasonably wonder whether the optimistic outlook from early series is skewed by reporting bias, with less favorable results unlikely to find their way into the literature. Larger series such as the National Cancer Institute studies from Lanza and colleagues [71] and Temeck and colleagues [68] report a 15% to 20% actuarial 5-year survival rate following pulmonary metastasectomy for Ewing's sarcoma.

Table 2
Results of pulmonary metastasectomy for Ewing's sarcoma

Reference	n	Survivors after metastasectomy
Richardson, 1961 [1]	3	2/3 alive at 5 y
Ridings, 1964 [72]	2	2/2 alive at 6 y and 11 y
Gronner and Sherman, 1970 [73]	1	1/1 dead at 49 mo
Ballantine et al, 1975 [4]	3	2/3 dead by 14 mo; 1 of 3 recurred at 6 mo
Rodgers et al, 1980 [25]	4	2/4 alive at 23 mo and 27 mo
Frenckner et al, 1982 [26]	1	1/1 alive at 9 y
Baldeyrou et al, 1984 [27]	14	Not specified
Lembke et al, 1986 [28]	4	3/4 alive at 6–51 mo
Lanza et al, 1987 [71]	10 Resectable	15% overall 5-y survival
	6 Unresectable	0% overall 5-y survival
Di Lorenzo and Collin, 1988 [29]	2	0/2 alive at 46 mo
Heij et al, 1994 [11]	12	0/12 alive at 5 y
Temeck et al, 1995 [68]	28	20% overall 5-y survival
Paulussen et al, 1998 [74]	20	35% 5-y event-free survival
Karnak et al, 2002 [32]	2	1/2 alive at 3 y
Briccoli et al, 2004 [75]	24	55% overall 5-y survival

The National Cancer Institute series by Lanza et al [71] draws a clear distinction between patients deemed to have "resectable" disease versus "unresectable" disease. The patients who had resectable disease had a range of 1 to 30 pulmonary nodules, and a 5-year actuarial survival rate of 15% was achieved. Those who had fewer than 4 nodules went on to have a longer disease-free interval before recurrence than those who had 4 or more nodules. Of the patients deemed unresectable at exploration, none survived for more than 22 months despite additional chemotherapy and radiotherapy. These results suggest that patients who have limited disease may have a better outcome than those who have more extensive disease, with the role of metastasectomy being potentially contributory. As the investigators stated, "it is not possible to determine from this retrospective review whether resectability indicates a more favorable prognosis or whether surgical resection influences outcome. It is likely that both biological properties of the tumor and successful reduction of tumor burden are important factors." These investigators also pointed out that 3 of 19 patients (16%) who had presumed metastases from Ewing's sarcoma turned out to have benign disease, so performance of the thoracotomy saved some patients from intensive systemic therapy after lung nodules had appeared.

A recent case-control study by Briccoli and colleagues [75] compared 24 patients who underwent metastasectomy with 34 patients matched for age, sex, tumor location, and disease-free interval but not matched for other treatments received. A survival benefit was reported at 5 years for those undergoing metastasectomy. The group receiving surgery, however, was a selected population, of whom half had only one pulmonary nodule to start with and did not have matched controls in this feature. The investigators concluded that lung metastasectomy should be "considered" in Ewing's sarcoma.

These reports must be counterbalanced against the continued evolution of chemotherapy and radiotherapy for Ewing's sarcoma. Retrospective reports from the German/European Intergroup Cooperative Ewing's Sarcoma Studies showed a benefit in event-free survival following whole-lung irradiation among patients who had primary metastatic Ewing's sarcoma to the lungs or pleura but showed no survival benefit among the small subset undergoing pulmonary resection [74,76].

There are technical difficulties inherent in the resection of Ewing's metastases. Tumors may be soft and fleshy, blending in with surrounding lung parenchyma. This characteristic makes them difficult to palpate and resect with negative margins, unlike the metastases from osteosarcoma, which tend to be firmer.

A reasonable policy toward pulmonary metastases of Ewing's sarcoma, therefore, is to operate to make a diagnosis and to consider complete resection only when disease is limited. Given the paucity of data in strong favor of surgery, however, pulmonary metastasectomy for this disease remains controversial. Chemotherapy and whole-lung irradiation are central components of the treatment of these patients.

Hepatoblastoma

Metastasectomy has been employed with favorable survival in selected patients who have hepatoblastoma. Enthusiasm for metastasectomy in this disease has been founded on case reports and small series. For example, Bradham and colleagues [77] reported on a "malignant hepatoma" resected from a 21-month-old girl in 1960 that was followed by a right pneumonectomy in 1961 for a large metastasis and a chest wall resection for recurrence that same year. The patient did well initially but succumbed 5 years later [78]. She had received radiotherapy but no chemotherapy. A 1995 report from Passmore and colleagues [79] described a boy who had a hepatoblastoma excised at age 14 months who underwent five thoracotomies for metastatic disease during the course of his childhood and was disease-free at age 12 years.

At the same time, it was observed that metastatic hepatoblastoma could also exhibit complete responses to chemotherapy. Among the 11 patients who had unresectable hepatoblastomas reported on by Pierro and colleagues [80] in 1989, 2 had lung metastases. The lung metastases completely disappeared in 1 of the 2 patients following preoperative chemotherapy. This finding was confirmed at autopsy (the patient exsanguinated during attempted resection of the primary liver tumor).

Further evidence that metastatic hepatoblastoma can be eradicated by chemotherapy came from a case reported by Dower and colleagues [81] in which a patient had disappearance of lung lesions with chemotherapy and then went on to undergo orthotopic liver transplantation to address the primary hepatoblastoma. Even with the consequent immunosuppression, lung metastases had not recurred in 38 months of follow-up.

Thus, a hybrid approach has developed for metastatic hepatoblastoma, with most centers favoring initial treatment with chemotherapy, followed by metastasectomy for lung lesions that respond incompletely. Two Japanese studies support this approach. The first is a case series by Uchiyama and colleagues [82]. Of their 19 patients whose primary hepatoblastomas were resectable, 9 had pulmonary metastases. All received chemotherapy, but the only survivors (of which there were 2 who had pulmonary metastases) were in the group that went on to have pulmonary metastasectomy. Matsunaga and colleagues [83] in 2003 similarly reported that the only survivors among 8 patients who had recurrent hepatoblastoma in the lungs were among the group receiving chemotherapy followed by surgical metastasectomy for each affected lung. In stage IV patients who had lung metastases at presentation, however, some patients treated with chemotherapy alone were long-term survivors; these were patients whose tumors displayed complete

radiographic disappearance. When residual metastases were present after chemotherapy, metastasectomy was performed.

Western studies support the Japanese reports. A Children's Cancer Group report described six stage I patients who progressed to pulmonary metastasis. Chemotherapy with or without metastasectomy did not cure every patient, but the only three long-term disease-free survivors (with follow-up ranging from 64 to 104 months) were in the group receiving chemotherapy followed by resection of the lung lesions [84]. Similar findings—that pulmonary metastatic spread could in some cases be eradicated by chemotherapy followed by surgery for residual disease—emerged from the trial by the International Society of Pediatric Oncology Liver Tumor Study Group [85,86].

Serum alpha fetoprotein is often a reliable marker with which to follow patients for recurrence. Black and colleagues [78] laid out several criteria for resection of pulmonary metastases of hepatoblastoma, among them that survival is enhanced when the alpha fetoprotein level demonstrates an initial drop following chemotherapy. The author has found this indicator particularly helpful: a drop in the alpha fetoprotein level indicates that an effective chemotherapy regimen has been identified and, even after complete metastasectomy is performed, the patient may receive adjuvant therapy with the same regimen to eliminate microscopic disease.

Differentiated thyroid cancer

Despite the lack of controlled prospective studies, ^{131}I has become the standard of care for treatment of children and adolescents who have lung metastases from differentiated thyroid cancer. Pulmonary metastasectomy is virtually absent in the literature among young patients who have this disease, except for isolated instances in which metastasectomy is pursued for diagnostic purposes only [27]. The rarity with which metastasectomy is pursued in this disease may be related to the tendency for disseminated thyroid cancer to present with miliary lung disease. In addition, the difficulty in establishing any role for surgical metastasectomy can be appreciated by understanding how low the mortality is to begin with for young patients who have disseminated thyroid cancer.

In a retrospective study requiring at least 10 years of follow-up, Vassilopoulou-Sellin and colleagues [87] reviewed 112 patients at M.D. Anderson Cancer Center who were diagnosed with differentiated thyroid cancer at age 19 years or younger. Ninety-nine of

112 patients were alive at last follow-up. Of the 13 who died, 6 died of progressive thyroid cancer at a mean duration of 26 years following initial diagnosis. Of the 6 who died of progressive thyroid cancer, 5 had lung metastases. A larger, multi-institutional cohort of pediatric patients compiled by Newman and co-workers [88] found only 2 disease-related deaths out of 329 patients. The 20-year progression-free survival rate after diagnosis was 60% (95% confidence interval: 54%–76%). Because mortality in this disease is so low and progression-free survival is so favorable for pediatric patients, the relative impact of any specific intervention on metastatic disease, whether it is metastasectomy or radioactive iodine treatment, is difficult to gauge [17].

As reported in the study by Newman and co-workers [88], 100% of the patients who had pulmonary metastases at diagnosis received radioactive iodine. Outcomes in this situation may be gleaned from two studies looking particularly at pediatric patients who had lung metastases from thyroid carcinoma. Nineteen patients in an M.D. Anderson Cancer Center cohort of 209 patients under age 25 years presented with pulmonary metastases [89]. Seventeen of these 19 patients had positive radio-iodine uptake scans in the lungs despite deceptively normal chest films in 8 patients. At a median follow-up of 4.5 years, no deaths had occurred, but scans had normalized for 6 of the 17 patients who had abnormal radioiodine uptake in the lungs following therapy with ^{131}I. Similarly, a Mayo Clinic study by Brink and colleagues [90] found that of 14 pediatric patients who had lung metastases from papillary thyroid cancer, all were alive at a mean follow-up of 19.3 years. Twelve of the 14 had received ^{131}I. Half of the 14 patients were alive with residual disease, but the other half had no evidence of disease. In these studies and others, the disappearance of metastatic disease has frequently been observed in association with the administration of radioactive iodine. Therefore, it remains the standard therapy.

Technical issues unique to pediatric patients

Anesthetic considerations

The author encourages patients to receive an epidural catheter for postoperative pain control. In infants and in children younger than 10 years, this catheter can usually be placed after general anesthesia has been induced. For older children and teenagers, the author has found that most anesthesiologists and pain management specialists are able to guide placement of the epidural with more confidence when the patient is awake, in a seated position, and able to describe paresthesias if they arise during epidural placement. By knowing what to expect in advance, most teenagers are willing to comply, and the resultant benefits seen in young patients' hospital stays due to improved postoperative deep breathing and coughing seem to outweigh the time and anxiety expended preoperatively.

Intraoperatively, single-lung ventilation is used whenever possible. Complete collapse of the lung in the operative field reduces the likelihood of a pulmonotomy when entering the pleural space and aids in the palpation of lung parenchyma for occult metastases. Accomplishing single-lung ventilation can be a challenge in pediatric patients; it is not possible in newborns and infants except by direct compression of the lung in the operative field. Commonly, hospitals stock 35 French double-lumen tubes, which are suitable for larger teenagers and older patients. Size 28 French double-lumen tubes exist but require the ready availability of a small enough flexible broncho-scope to position them. Typically, therefore, children younger than teenagers are too small for effective placement and ventilation with a double-lumen endo-tracheal tube.

In these situations, a bronchial blocker is sometimes used (Fig. 6). The author uses Fogarty balloon catheters for this purpose. The blocker must be threaded down the trachea in parallel with the endotracheal tube, and a flexible fiberoptic broncho-scope is passed down the endotracheal tube to visualize positioning of the blocker. The size of the balloon must be noted, because even when deflated, it may be so large that it completely occludes a pediatric bronchus. If the surgeon wants to manually expel the air from the operative lung at the beginning of the surgery or to temporarily reinflate the lung at the end

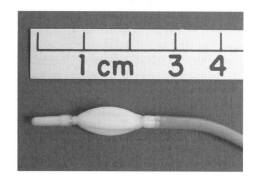

Fig. 6. An 8 French bronchial blocker. The balloon size, even when deflated, poses the risk of complete occlusion of a pediatric main-stem bronchus if the child is small enough.

of the surgery to check for air leaks, then these maneuvers will be hampered by a balloon that is too large when deflated. This situation can be appreciated from Fig. 6. If a bronchial blocker cannot be suitably used, the next best choice is a right or left main-stem intubation.

Bronchoscopy and lymph node dissection

Bronchoscopy by the surgeon has usually not been the author's practice in advance of metastasectomy. Because pediatric tumors are not epithelial malignancies originating in the bronchial tree but are usually peripheral masses in the parenchyma, bronchoscopy is usually noncontributory and reserved for special instances such as making a decision as to whether a centrally located mass may require lobectomy due to impingement on a secondary bronchus. Hilar lymph node dissection, another routine staple of adult thoracic surgery, has not been routine unless gross involvement of nodes is found, which can occasionally occur with osteosarcoma, hepatoblastoma, or Wilms tumor.

Muscle-sparing approach to thoracotomy

The author employs a muscle-sparing approach whenever possible in pediatric patients. Avoidance of sectioning the latissimus muscle seems to result in a substantial difference in postoperative pain, and for some patients who have primary tumors of the limbs, this technique preserves the latissimus for future flap reconstructions that may be critical for the patient's outcome. In the author's experience at Memorial Sloan-Kettering Cancer Center, patients have frequently been comfortable enough on oral pain medication to be successfully discharged within 72 hours of a full thoracotomy when the muscle-sparing approach has been used. This technique has been so well-tolerated by patients that the author performs staged bilateral thoracotomies (with the resulting advantages in the ability to palpate all segments of the lung, including the left lower lobe) rather than median sternotomy when there is a question about bilateral lesions.

To employ this method, the patient is placed in the standard lateral decubitus position, and the skin incision is a standard posterolateral thoracotomy incision (Fig. 7). The triangle of auscultation is identified, marked by the latissimus inferiorly, the trapezius medially, and the rhomboid and serratus muscles laterally (Fig. 8). Rather than cutting any muscle fibers, the surgeon bluntly elevates these muscles by dissection in the areolar plane between muscle and

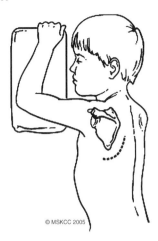

© MSKCC 2005

Fig. 7. Position and skin incision for a muscle-sparing thoracotomy in a pediatric patient. (Courtesy of Memorial Sloan-Kettering Cancer Center, New York, New York; with permission.)

ribcage. A space is developed just large enough to admit the surgeon's hand. This opening may at first seem to be only a small opening into the thorax; however, the author has found that the combination of the compliance of the pediatric chest wall plus the use of of pharmacologic muscle relaxation enables the development of an ample thoracotomy using this approach if one is patient and expands the Finochietto rib spreaders a little at a time. When necessary, a rib is divided, but a rib segment is not removed.

Sewing versus stapling

After the lung is deflated, inspected, and palpated, metastases are removed using surgical staplers or by freehand using the precision cautery technique [91], with suture closure of the pulmonotomy. Avoiding the placement of staples may, in theory, leave fewer dense objects in the lung that will confound attempts to palpate the lung during future thoracotomies; however, neither technique is failsafe: the author had a case of thoracotomy for recurrent osteosarcoma in which a "nodule" palpated by the surgeon proved, on pathologic sectioning, to be a suture placed 1 year earlier. When metastases are removed with the pinpoint cautery technique, the author's present practice is to close the resulting pulmonotomy using a bidirectional running locked suture of 2-0 or 3-0 polydioxanone, taking care to obliterate the dead space.

When a surgical stapler is employed, stapler choices may be different for pediatric patients than for adults in corresponding situations, and attention

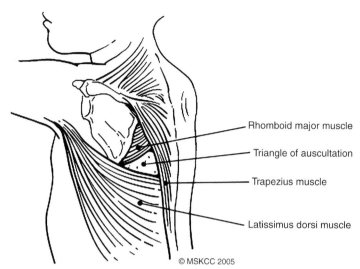

© MSKCC 2005

Rhomboid major muscle

Triangle of auscultation

Trapezius muscle

Latissimus dorsi muscle

Fig. 8. The triangle of auscultation. The areolar tissue bounded by latissimus, trapezius, rhomboid, and (inserting into the inferior border of the scapula and not shown) serratus anterior muscles is bluntly spread to expose the underlying ribcage. (Courtesy of Memorial Sloan-Kettering Cancer Center, New York, New York; with permission.)

to this difference can minimize or eradicate post-operative air leaks. It should be remembered that the different sizes for available staple cartridges reflect variations in the height (not the length) of the staples, and hence, the choice of staple cartridge is dictated by the thickness of the pulmonary parenchyma to be stapled (Fig. 9). For instance, 2.5-mm cartridges are well suited for sealing a peripheral wedge resection in a pediatric patient; 3.5-mm cartridges are appropriate for thicker or inflamed tissue or for closing a bronchus in an older child; and 4.8-mm cartridges should be reserved for more central wedge resections

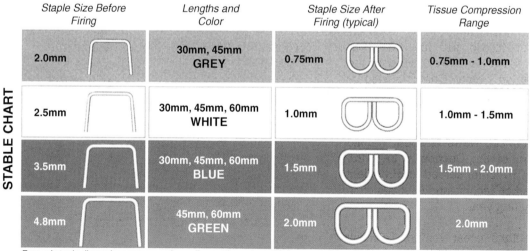

STABLE CHART

Staple Size Before Firing	Lengths and Color	Staple Size After Firing (typical)	Tissue Compression Range
2.0mm	30mm, 45mm GREY	0.75mm	0.75mm - 1.0mm
2.5mm	30mm, 45mm, 60mm WHITE	1.0mm	1.0mm - 1.5mm
3.5mm	30mm, 45mm, 60mm BLUE	1.5mm	1.5mm - 2.0mm
4.8mm	45mm, 60mm GREEN	2.0mm	2.0mm

Formed staple dimensions may vary depending on tissue type, thickness, and density.
Please refer to package insert for complete instructions, warnings, precautions and contraindications.

Fig. 9. Diagram of commonly available sizes for disposable surgical staplers. Note that the differences among stapler cartridges reflect differences predominantly in staple height, not in the distance between clips. Peripheral wedge resections in children are most effectively performed with 2.5- or 3.5-mm staples, enabling airtight closure of typical tissue thicknesses encountered in pediatric patients. (Courtesy of Jeffrey Erickson. Copyright © 2005 United States Surgical, a division of Tyco Healthcare Group LP. All rights reserved. Reprinted with the permission of United States Surgical, a division of Tyco Healthcare Group LP.)

that require traversing a thick layer of parenchyma. The author's colleagues who operate on adults rely heavily on the 4.8-mm cartridges, but these will result in air leakage in some pediatric settings.

References

[1] Richardson WR. Progress in pediatric cancer surgery. Arch Surg 1961;82:641–55.

[2] White JF, Krivit W. Surgical excision of pulmonary metastases. Pediatrics 1962;29:927–32.

[3] Cliffton EE, Pool JL. Treatment of lung metastases in children with combined therapy: surgery and/or irradiation and chemotherapy. J Thorac Cardiovasc Surg 1967;54(3):403–21.

[4] Ballantine TVN, Wiseman NE, Filler RM. Assessment of pulmonary wedge resection for the treatment of lung metastases. J Pediatr Surg 1975;10(5):671–6.

[5] Kilman JW, Kronenberg MW, O'Neill JA, et al. Surgical resection for pulmonary metastases in children. Arch Surg 1969;99:158–65.

[6] Martini N, Huvos AG, Miké V, et al. Multiple pulmonary resections in the treatment of osteogenic sarcoma. Ann Thorac Surg 1971;12:271–80.

[7] Marcove RC, Miké V, Hajek JV, et al. Osteogenic sarcoma under the age of twenty-one: a review of one hundred and forty-five operative cases. J Bone Joint Surg Am 1970;52(3):411–23.

[8] Beattie EJ, Harvey JC, Marcove R, et al. Results of multiple pulmonary resections for metastatic osteogenic sarcoma after two decades. J Surg Oncol 1991; 46:154–5.

[9] Barrows G, Kmetz DR. Treatment of lobar pulmonary metastasis in childhood cancer. J Ky Med Assoc 1975; 73(3):367–70.

[10] Torre W, Rodriguez-Spiteri N, Sierrasesumaga L. Current role for resection of thoracic metastases in children and young adults—do we need different strategies for this population? Thorac Cardiov Surg 2004; 52:90–5.

[11] Heij HA, Vos A, de Kraker J, et al. Prognostic factors in surgery for pulmonary metastases in children. Surgery 1994;115:687–93.

[12] Chang AE, Schaner EG, Conkle DM, et al. Evaluation of computed tomography in the detection of pulmonary metastases: a prospective study. Cancer 1979;43: 913–6.

[13] Green DM. Wilms' tumour. Eur J Cancer 1997;33: 409–18.

[14] Wilimas JA, Douglass EC, Magill HL, et al. Significance of pulmonary computed tomography at diagnosis in Wilms' tumor. J Clin Oncol 1988;6:1144–6.

[15] Meisel JA, Guthrie KA, Breslow NE, et al. Significance and management of computed tomography detected pulmonary nodules: a report from the National Wilms Tumor Study Group. Int J Radiat Oncol Biol Phys 1999;44:579–85.

[16] Green DM. Use of chest computed tomography for staging and treatment of Wilms' tumor in children. J Clin Oncol 2002;20:2763–4.

[17] Yeh SDJ, La Quaglia MP. [131]I therapy for pediatric thyroid cancer. Semin Pediatr Surg 1997;6(3):128–33.

[18] Rosenfield NS, Keller MS, Markowitz RI, et al. CT differentiation of benign and malignant lung nodules in children. J Pediatr Surg 1992;27:459–61.

[19] McCarville MB, Kaste SC, Cain AM, et al. Prognostic factors and imaging patterns of recurrent pulmonary nodules after thoracotomy in children with osteosarcoma. Cancer 2001;91:1170–6.

[20] Hardaway BW, Hoffer FA, Rao BN. Needle localization of small pediatric tumors for surgical biopsy. Pediatr Radiol 2000;30:318–22.

[21] Waldhausen JHT, Shaw DWW, Hall DG, et al. Needle localization for thoracoscopic resection of small pulmonary nodules in children. J Pediatr Surg 1997;32: 1624–5.

[22] Partrick DA, Bensard DD, Teitelbaum DH, et al. Successful thoracoscopic lung biopsy in children utilizing preoperative CT-guided localization. J Pediatr Surg 2002;37:970–3.

[23] Scorpio RJ, Stokes K, Grattan-Smith D, et al. Percutaneous localization of small pulmonary metastases, enabling limited resection. J Pediatr Surg 1994;29: 685–7.

[24] McConnell PI, Feola GP, Meyers RL. Methylene blue-stained autologous blood for needle localization and thoracoscopic resection of deep pulmonary nodules. J Pediatr Surg 2002;37:1729–31.

[25] Rodgers BM, Talbert JL, Alexander JA. Pulmonary metastases in childhood sarcoma. Ann Thorac Surg 1980;29:410–4.

[26] Frenckner B, Lännergren K, Söderlund S. Results of surgical treatment of lung metastases in children. Scand J Thor Cardiovasc Surg 1982;16:201–4.

[27] Baldeyrou P, Lemoine G, Zucker JM, et al. Pulmonary metastases in children: the place of surgery. J Pediatr Surg 1984;19:121–5.

[28] Lembke J, Havers W, Doetsch N, et al. Long-term results following surgical removal of pulmonary metastases in children with malignomas. Thorac Cardiovasc Surg 1986;34:137–9.

[29] Di Lorenzo M, Collin P-P. Pulmonary metastases in children: results of surgical treatment. J Pediatr Surg 1988;23(8):762–5.

[30] de Kraker J, Lemerle J, Voûte PA, et al. Wilms' tumor with pulmonary metastases at diagnosis: the significance of primary chemotherapy. J Clin Oncol 1990;8: 1187–90.

[31] Green DM, Breslow NE, Ii Y, et al. The role of surgical excision in the management of relapsed Wilms' tumor patients with pulmonary metastases: a report from the National Wilms' Tumor Study. J Pediatr Surg 1991;26: 728–33.

[32] Karnak I, Emin Senocak ME, Kutluk T, et al. Pulmonary metastases in children: an analysis of surgical spectrum. Eur J Pediatr Surg 2002;12:151–8.

[33] Abel RM, Brown J, Moreland B, et al. Pulmonary metastasectomy for pediatric solid tumors. Pediatr Surg Int 2004;20:630–2.

[34] Bond JV, Martin EC. Pulmonary metastases in Wilms' tumor. Clin Radiol 1976;27:191–5.

[35] Green DM, Finklestein JZ, Tefft ME, et al. Diffuse interstitial pneumonitis after pulmonary irradiation for metastatic Wilms' tumor. Cancer 1989;63:450–3.

[36] Green DM, Breslow NE, Beckwith JB, et al. Comparison between single-dose and divided-dose administration of dactinomycin and doxorubicin for patients with Wilms' tumor: a report from the National Wilms' Tumor Study Group. J Clin Oncol 1998;16: 237–45.

[37] Green DM, Beckwith JB, Breslow NE, et al. Treatment of children with stages II to IV anaplastic Wilms' tumor: a report from the National Wilms' Tumor Study Group. J Clin Oncol 1994;12:2126–31.

[38] Cowie F, Corbett R, Pinkerton CR. Lung involvement in neuroblastoma: incidence and characteristics. Med Pediatr Oncol 1997;28:429–32.

[39] DuBois SG, Kalika Y, Lukens JN, et al. Metastatic sites in stage IV and IVS neuroblastoma correlate with age, tumor biology, and survival. J Pediatr Hematol Oncol 1999;21(3):181–9.

[40] Kammen BF, Matthay KK, Pacharn P, et al. Pulmonary metastases at diagnosis of neuroblastoma in pediatric patients: CT findings and prognosis. AJR Am J Roentgenol 2001;176(3):755–9.

[41] Baka M, Pourtsidis A, Bouhoutsou D, et al. Neuroblastoma metastatic to the lungs at diagnosis. Med Pediatr Oncol 2003;41(2):147–9.

[42] Cohn K, Gottesman L, Brennan M. Adrenocortical carcinoma. Surgery 1986;100(6):1170–7.

[43] Schulick RD, Brennan MF. Long-term survival after complete resection and repeat resection in patients with adrenocortical carcinoma. Ann Surg Oncol 1999;6(8): 719–26.

[44] Kwauk S, Burt M. Pulmonary metastases from adrenal cortical carcinoma: results of resection. J Surg Oncol 1993;53:243–6.

[45] Jensen JC, Pass HI, Sindelar WF, et al. Recurrent or metastatic disease in select patients with adrenocortical carcinoma. Arch Surg 1991;126:457–61.

[46] De León DD, Lange BJ, Walterhouse D, et al. Long-term (15 years) outcome in an infant with metastatic adrenocortical carcinoma. J Clin Endocrinol Metab 2002;87:4452–6.

[47] Appelqvist P, Kostiainen S. Multiple thoracotomy combined with chemotherapy in metastatic adrenal cortical carcinoma: a case report and review of the literature. J Surg Oncol 1983;24:1–4.

[48] Sandrini R, Ribeiro RC, DeLacerda L. Childhood adrenocortical tumors. J Clin Endocrinol Metab 1997; 82(7):2027–31.

[49] Ribeiro RC, Michalkiewicz EL, Figueiredo BC, et al. Adrenocortical tumors in children. Braz J Med Bio Res 2000;33(10):1225–34.

[50] Hankins FD, DeSanto DA. Treatment of osteogenic sarcoma that had metastasized to the lungs: 25-year survival of a patient. West J Med 1980;132(3):245–8.

[51] Schaller RT, Haas J, Schaller J, et al. Improved survival in children with osteosarcoma following resection of pulmonary metastases. J Pediatr Surg 1982;17:546–50.

[52] Goorin AM, Delorey MJ, Lack EE, et al. Prognostic significance of complete surgical resection of pulmonary metastases in patients with osteogenic sarcoma: analysis of 32 patients. J Clin Oncol 1984;2:425–31.

[53] Meyers PA, Heller G, Healey JH, et al. Osteogenic sarcoma with clinically detectable metastasis at initial presentation. J Clin Oncol 1993;11:449–53.

[54] Kager L, Zoubek A, Pötschger U, et al. Primary metastatic osteosarcoma: presentation and outcome of patients treated on neoadjuvant cooperative osteosarcoma study group protocols. J Clin Oncol 2003;21:2011–8.

[55] Temeck BK, Wexler LH, Steinberg SM, et al. Reoperative pulmonary metastasectomy for sarcomatous pediatric histologies. Ann Thorac Surg 1998;66: 908–13.

[56] Jaffe N, Carrasco H, Raymond K, et al. Can cure in patients with osteosarcoma be achieved exclusively with chemotherapy and abrogation of surgery? Cancer 2002;95:2202–10.

[57] Kayton ML, Huvos AG, Casher J, et al. Computed tomographic scan of the chest underestimates the number of metastatic lesions in osteosarcoma. J Pediatr Surg 2006;41:200–6.

[58] Su WT, Chewning J, Abramson S, et al. Surgical management and outcome of osteosarcoma patients with unilateral pulmonary metastases. J Pediatr Surg 2004;39:418–23.

[59] Dillon P, Maurer H, Jenkins J, et al. A prospective study of nonrhabdomyosarcoma soft tissue sarcomas in the pediatric age group. J Pediatr Surg 1992;27:241–5.

[60] Andrassy RJ, Okcu MF, Despa S, et al. Synovial sarcoma in children: surgical lessons from a single institution and review of the literature. J Am Coll Surg 2001;192:305–13.

[61] Pappo AS, Rao BN, Jenkins JJ, et al. Metastatic nonrhabdomyosarcomatous soft-tissue sarcomas in children and adolescents: the St. Jude Children's Research Hospital experience. Med Pediatr Oncol 1999;33: 76–82.

[62] Pappo AS, Fontanesi J, Luo X, et al. Synovial sarcoma in children and adolescents: the St Jude Children's Research Hospital experience. J Clin Oncol 1994;12: 2360–6.

[63] Lieberman PH, Brennan MF, Kimmel M, et al. Alveolar soft-part sarcoma: a clinico-pathologic study of half a century. Cancer 1989;63:1–13.

[64] Portera CA, Ho V, Patel SR, et al. Alveolar soft part sarcoma: clinical course and patterns of metastasis in 70 patients treated at a single institution. Cancer 2001; 91:585–91.

[65] Casanova M, Ferrari A, Bisogno G, et al. Alveolar soft part sarcoma in children and adolescents: a report from the Soft-Tissue Sarcoma Italian Cooperative Group. Ann Oncol 2000;11:1445–9.

[66] Pappo AS, Parham DM, Cain A, et al. Alveolar soft part sarcoma in children and adolescents: clinical features and outcome of 11 patients. Med Pediatr Oncol 1996;26:81–4.

[67] Kayton ML, Meyers P, Wexler LH, et al. Clinical presentation, treatment, and outcome of alveolar soft part sarcoma in children, adolescents, and young adults. J Pediatr Surg 2006;41:187–93.

[68] Temeck BK, Wexler LH, Steinberg SM, et al. Metastasectomy for sarcomatous pediatric histologies: results and prognostic factors. Ann Thorac Surg 1995; 59:1385–90.

[69] Rodeberg D, Arndt C, Breneman J, et al. Characteristics and outcomes of rhabdomyosarcoma patients with isolated lung metastases from IRS-IV. J Pediatr Surg 2005;40:256–62.

[70] Meyers PA, Levy AS. Ewing's sarcoma. Curr Treat Options Oncol 2000;1(3):247–57.

[71] Lanza LA, Miser JS, Pass HI, et al. The role of resection in the treatment of pulmonary metastases from Ewing's sarcoma. J Thorac Cardiovasc Surg 1987;94: 181–7.

[72] Ridings GR. Ewing's tumor. Radiol Clin North Am 1964;50:315–25.

[73] Gronner AT, Sherman RS. Eight-year-survival in a patient with Ewing's sarcoma of the fibula metastatic to the lung. Oncology 1970;24(3):230–9.

[74] Paulussen M, Ahrens S, Craft AW, et al. Ewing's tumors with primary lung metastases: survival analysis of 114 (European Intergroup) Cooperative Ewing's Sarcoma Studies patients. J Clin Oncol 1998;16:3044–52.

[75] Briccoli A, Rocca M, Ferrari S, et al. Surgery for lung metastases in Ewing's sarcoma of bone. Eur J Surg Oncol 2004;30(1):63–7.

[76] Paulussen M, Ahrens S, Burdach S, et al. Primary metastatic (stage IV) Ewing tumor: survival analysis of 171 patients from the EICESS studies. Ann Oncol 1998;9:275–81.

[77] Bradham RR, Paul JR, Thrower WB, et al. Malignant hepatoma in a child: survival following right hepatectomy, right pneumonectomy, and resection of diaphragmatic and parietal recurrence. Surgery 1965;57:767–73.

[78] Black CT, Luck SR, Musemeche CA, et al. Aggressive excision of pulmonary metastases is warranted in the management of childhood hepatic tumors. J Pediatr Surg 1991;26:1082–6.

[79] Passmore SJ, Noblett HR, Wisheart JD, et al. Prolonged survival following multiple thoracotomies for metastatic hepatoblastoma. Med Pediatr Oncol 1995; 24:58–60.

[80] Pierro A, Langevin AM, Filler RM, et al. Preoperative chemotherapy in "unresectable" hepatoblastoma. J Pediatr Surg 1989;24:24–9.

[81] Dower NA, Smith LJ, Lees G, et al. Experience with aggressive therapy in three children with unresectable malignant liver tumors. Med Pediatr Oncol 2000;34: 132–5.

[82] Uchiyama M, Iwafuchi M, Naito M, et al. A study of therapy for pediatric hepatoblastoma: prevention and treatment of pulmonary metastasis. Eur J Pediatr Surg 1999;9:142–5.

[83] Matsunaga T, Sasaki F, Ohira M, et al. Analysis of treatment outcome for children with recurrent or metastatic hepatoblastoma. Pediatr Surg Int 2003;19: 142–6.

[84] Feusner JH, Krailo MD, Haas JE, et al. Treatment of pulmonary metastases of initial stage I hepatoblastoma in childhood. Cancer 1993;71:859–64.

[85] Perilongo G, Brown J, Shafford E, et al. Hepatoblastoma presenting with lung metastases. Cancer 2000; 89:1845–53.

[86] Schnater JM, Aronson DC, Plaschkes J, et al. Surgical view of the treatment of patients with hepatoblastoma. Cancer 2002;94:1111–20.

[87] Vassilopoulou-Sellin R, Goepfert H, Raney B, et al. Differentiated thyroid cancer in children and adolescents: clinical outcome and mortality after long-term follow-up. Head Neck 1998;20:549–55.

[88] Newman KD, Black T, Heller G, et al. Differentiated thyroid cancer: determinants of disease progression in patients <21 years of age at diagnosis. Ann Surg 1998; 227(4):533–41.

[89] Vassilopoulou-Sellin R, Klein MJ, Smith TH, et al. Pulmonary metastases in children and young adults with differentiated thyroid cancer. Cancer 1993;71: 1348–52.

[90] Brink JS, van Heerden JA, McIver B, et al. Papillary thyroid cancer with pulmonary metastases in children: long-term prognosis. Surgery 2000;128:881–7.

[91] Cooper JD, Perelman M, Todd TRJ, et al. Precision cautery excision of pulmonary lesions. Ann Thorac Surg 1986;41:51–3.

ELSEVIER
SAUNDERS

Thorac Surg Clin 16 (2006) 185 – 198

THORACIC
SURGERY
CLINICS

Isolated Lung Perfusion for Pulmonary Metastases

Jeroen M.H. Hendriks, MD, PhD[a],*, Bart P. Van Putte, MD, PhD[b],
Marco Grootenboers, MD[b], Wim J. Van Boven, MD[b],
Franz Schramel, MD, PhD[b], Paul E.Y. Van Schil, MD, PhD[a]

[a]Department of Thoracic and Vascular Surgery, University Hospital Antwerp, Wilrijkstraat 10 B-2650, Edegem, Belgium
[b]Department of Pulmonary Medicine and Surgery, Antonius Hospital, Koekoekslaan I, 3435 CM Nieuwegein, The Netherlands

The efficacy of intravenous chemotherapy for patients with metastatic malignant disease is limited by systemic toxicity and so far has not resulted in a significant prolongation of survival. Response rates of only 25% to 50% are seen and the duration of benefit is usually short-lived. When lung metastases are unresectable, most patients die within 1 year, and for the highly selected group of patients with resectable lung metastases, 5-year survival rates of only 20% to 40% after complete surgical resection have been achieved [2] because even after an apparently complete resection, most patients experience recurrent pulmonary disease from undetected micrometastatic disease present at the time of surgery.

Isolated lung perfusion (ILuP) is a surgical technique developed to allow the delivery of high-dose chemotherapy to the lung with minimal systemic exposure to improve first-order targeting [1] (Table 1). This technique allows delivery of a biologic agent to the lung in high doses by the pulmonary artery while the pulmonary venous effluent is diverted, minimizing systemic exposure such that no metabolism takes place in the liver or kidneys. Although ILuP was originally developed to convert unresectable pulmonary metastatic disease into resectable disease, several more recent studies have focused on patients with resectable disease with the goal of eliminating micro-

metastatic disease [2]. In this chapter, we consider the development of animal models of ILuP and then review the available information regarding the agents that can be delivered by this technique.

The concept of isolated organ perfusion was initiated in 1958 by Creech, who tested nitrogen mustard in different organs, such as the extremities and the lungs [3]. Since the 1960s, most research involving isolated organ perfusion has been with extremities for melanoma and sarcoma, with impressive response rates approaching 100% [4]. Research into ILuP was begun in 1983 by Johnston and collaborators, who focused on the feasibility of staged bilateral isolated single-lung perfusion and simultaneous bilateral lung perfusion in both dogs and humans (Fig. 1). Johnston was a pioneer in the field of thoracic surgery [5], addressing the areas of the pharmacokinetics of doxorubicin [6,7], the toxicity of ILuP with doxorubicin [6,8], the effect of hyperthermia on normal lungs, and the effect of hyperthermia on the uptake of doxorubicin by the lungs during ILuP [9,10]. The lung proved to be an ideal organ for ILuP because it is symmetrical, with an arterial supply that is almost exclusively from the pulmonary artery and complete venous drainage into the two pulmonary veins. Further, at thoracotomy, the pulmonary vasculature is readily accessible. Finally, the lung can tolerate an impressive 44.4°C for 2 hours without significantly impact on physiologic variables [11,12].

Current phase I trials with ILuP have been designed using staged bilateral thoracotomies separated by an interval of 4 to 6 weeks [13–16]. If an extracorporeal circuit is used, both lungs can be per-

* Corresponding author.

E-mail address: jeroen.hendriks@uza.be
(J.M.H. Hendriks).

Table 1
Methods of first-order targeting

Biochemical	Enzyme binding
	Receptor binding
	Antibody trapping
Biophysical	Embolic trapping
	Inhalation
	Altered microvascular barriers
	Regional infusion
	Isolated perfusion
Bioadhesion	Combined biophysical and biochemical

From Johnston MR. Lung perfusion and other methods of targeting therapy to lung tumors. Chest Surg Clin North Am 1995;5:139–56; with permission.

fused simultaneously but this technique has not been adopted, because to place the extracorporeal circuit, a larger incision such as a clamshell thoracotomy is required, which combined with bilateral metastasectomy results in a more complex procedure and asso-

ciated increased morbidity. A systemic leakage of the perfusate, which is difficult to control in cases of isolated limb or isolated liver perfusion because of multiple veins draining the organ, has proven more readily controlled during ILuP as the bronchial artery circulation drains almost exclusively to the pulmonary veins. In addition, ILuP may be expected to be more effective in the treatment of pulmonary metastases as these receive most of their blood from the pulmonary circulation [17,18] in contrast to lung cancer in which a dual circulation by both the pulmonary and bronchial circulation is present [19]. Since the initiation of research by the group of Johnston, several groups in the USA, Europe, and Japan have developed models of lung metastases that have been used to test the efficacy of ILuP when used to administer different chemotherapeutic agents active against sarcoma, carcinoma, and melanoma. By 2005, several phase I clinical studies of ILuP have

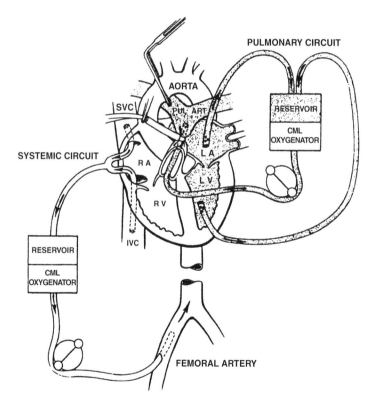

Fig. 1. Bilateral isolated lung perfusion circuit. The pulmonary artery is composed of a left atrial and a left ventricular gravity drainage system and perfusion is to the main pulmonary artery. The systemic circuit drains blood from the superior and inferior vena cava and perfuses oxygenated blood to the femoral artery. Note that the aorta is cross-clamped to prevent coronary blood flow and mixing of the pulmonary and systemic circulation. Another option could be the insertion of a coronary sinus cannula to drain the coronary circulation without cross-clamping the aorta. (*From* Johnston MR, Christensen CW, Minchin RF, et al. Isolated total lung perfusion as a means to deliver organ-specific chemotherapy: long-term studies in animals. Surgery 1985; 98:35–44; with permission.)

been completed and a phase II study of ILuP with melphalan is planned.

Models of isolated lung perfusion

Since the first ILuP experiments in 1983, large animals like pigs and dogs have been used to explore drug pharmacokinetics as preparation for human studies [5]. Because of a lack of an animal tumor model, only technical and pharmacokinetic questions have been answered and an evaluation of the anti-neoplastic efficacy of ILuP has not been performed. The ideal chemotherapeutic agent for ILuP would be rapidly taken-up out of the blood stream, preferably into tumor tissue rather than lung tissue, and would be without pulmonary toxicity at dose levels that are significantly higher than for intravenous therapy and without leakage back in to the pulmonary circulation after ILuP is completed. The drug's effect should be rapid because most ILuP treatments have been limited to 90 minutes in an attempt to minimize lung edema and tissue hypoxia. The ILuP circuits used in

large animals experiments have by and large been transferred to the clinical situation for phase I studies, but many differences regarding the circuit used exist between research groups. Most surgeons prefer a lateral thoracotomy, although a sternotomy has been used. Recently, video-assisted thoracic surgical (VATS) techniques for ILuP have been described [20]. Two different perfusion techniques for ILuP have been described: a single pass system (SP), which discards the venous effluent after one passage through the lung [21], and a recirculating blood circuit (RB), which collects the venous effluent into a closed circuit that consists of a roller pump, a cardiotomy reservoir, a heat exchanger, and blood filter (Fig. 2), and re-delivers it into the lung. An oxygenator is incorporated in this closed circuit in most large animal models [21–23], but no hypoxic complications have been seen without an oxygenator [5,9] as long as the lungs are ventilated during ILuP and the duration of perfusion limited. In SP ILuP, drug kinetic studies ensure a constant concentration in the perfusate facilitating drug kinetic studies, but large amounts of costly perfusate and drugs are needed. Therefore, SP

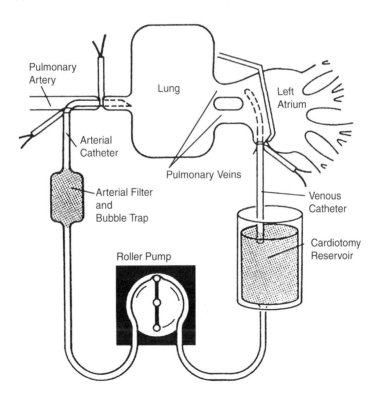

Fig. 2. Isolated lung perfusion circuit used in animal and human experiments. The left atrium is drained by gravity, and a roller pump is used to perfusate the left lung through the left pulmonary artery. A bubble trap and filter prevent clots and air from entering the pulmonary circulation. (*From* Johnston MR, Minchin R, Shull JH, et al. Isolated lung perfusion with adriamycin. A preclinical study. Cancer 1983;52:404–9; with permission.)

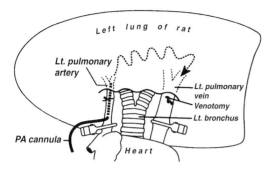

Fig. 3. Left isolated lung perfusion in the rat. (*From* Nawata S, Abolhada A, Ross H, et al. Sequential bilateral isolated lung perfusion in the rat: an experimental model. Ann Thorac Surg 1997;63:796–9; with permission.)

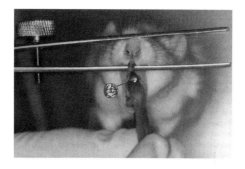

Fig. 5. After retracting the tongue, the vocal cords become visible by looking downward into the animal's pharynx. (*From* Hendriks J, Van Schil P, Eyskens E. Modified technique of isolated left lung perfusion in the rate. Eur Surg Res 1999;31:93–6; with permission.)

ILuP has been only rarely used in large animal studies and clinical practice. Although the standard ILuP technique in clinical trials has been antegrade perfusion through the pulmonary artery while the effluens is collected at the venous site [5], retrograde ILuP by the pulmonary veins has been introduced since 2002 as an alternative technique [23].

Although a large animal tumor model has not been developed, during the early 1990s researchers at Memorial Sloan-Kettering Cancer Center developed a rat model of ILuP to investigate anti-neoplastic efficacy [24] (Fig. 3). Different modifications of the original model have been made to the specific technique of ILuP [25,26] and of intubation with mechanical ventilation [26] (Figs. 4–6). The standard technique was SP ILuP [24], but RB ILuP [27] and

retrograde ILuP in a rat model have been tested successfully [28,29]. Because the left lung of the Fisher and Wag/Rij rat is unilobar with a long segment of extrapericardial pulmonary artery and vein (Fig. 7), ILuP was initially developed for the left lung [24,26], but more recently sequential bilateral ILuP in the rat has been described [30]. For toxicity studies, a contralateral right pneumonectomy is performed after a recovery period to demonstrate that the treated left lung functions [31]. For tumor efficacy studies, models for metastatic sarcoma and colorectal disease were developed and tested for reproducibility [32–34]. In general, single cell suspensions of viable tumor cells are injected into the femoral vein. Approximately 1 week after tumor inoculation, left ILuP with the study drug is performed. Two to 3 weeks later, the

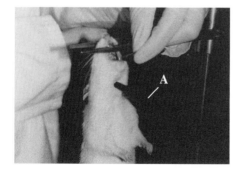

Fig. 4. A rat is hung up by his upper incisor teeth in a vertical supine position. A=cold light source. (*From* Hendriks J, Van Schil P, Eyskens E. Modified technique of isolated left lung perfusion in the rate. Eur Surg Res 1999;31:93–6; with permission.)

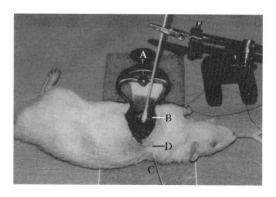

Fig. 6. Instead of the revised technique by Wang, retractor (*A*) and lung (*B*) are positioned anteriorly and the PE-10 catheter (*C*) is introduced into the chest through a 16-gauge Angiocath (*D*). (*From* Hendriks J, Van Schil P, Eyskens E. Modified technique of isolated left lung perfusion in the rate. Eur Surg Res 1999;31:93–6; with permission.)

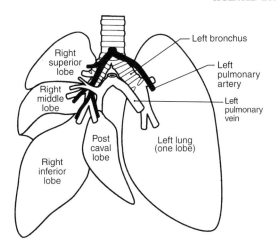

Fig. 7. Anatomy of Fisher 344 rat lungs. The right lung is composed of four lobes, and the left lung is a unilobar structure (*From* Nawata S, Abolhada A, Ross H, et al. Sequential bilateral isolated lung perfusion in the rat: an experimental model. Ann Thorac Surg 1997;63:796–9; with permission.)

rats are sacrificed, and lung blocks are stained black with India ink according to the technique of Wexler [35], and tumor nodules are counted [32,34]. The left treated lung can be compared with the right untreated side or comparisons can be made between rats. For survival studies, a rat model of unilateral lung metastases was developed [36]. Single tumor cells were injected into the left pulmonary artery while the right pulmonary artery is temporarily occluded, leading to left lung metastases only. After ILuP of the diseased lung is performed, survival was recorded without the variability in observations because of the risk of death caused by disease in the right lung. A unique model of ex vivo human ILuP was developed by Linder and colleagues in 1996 [37]. Human lungs that were resected for stage I and stage II non-small cell lung cancer were attached to an ex vivo isolated lung perfusion circuit similar to the one used for clinical studies of ILuP. The immediate advantage of this model is to study pharmacokinetic parameters in a human lung block while eliminating the need to perform such studies in animals like rats, pigs, or dogs. A similar model is currently being used at our hospital for pharmacokinetic experiments with melphalan and gemcitabine.

Tumor necrosis factor alpha

Since 1994, the pharmacokinetics and efficacy of ILuP with the biological response modifier tumor necrosis factor alpha (TNFα) has been studied exten-

sively in rat and pig models [22,32,34]. These studies have demonstrated that TNFα is an excellent agent for use in isolated organ perfusion for two reasons. First, the dose required for antitumor effects is 200 to 400 μg/kg body weight, which is far more than the maximally tolerable intravenous dose of 5 to 10 μg/kg, which has poor anti-tumor effect [38]. Second, the effect of a single exposure of the lung to TNFα administered by ILuP is impressive, with destruction of bulky tumors within 30 minutes, which is similar to results seen with isolated limb perfusion with TNFα for melanoma and sarcoma [4]. When rats with lung sarcoma metastases were perfused with 420 μg of murine TNFα or with recombinant human TNFα, significantly less tumor nodules were found in the treated left lung than in the unperfused right lung [39]. The same group also investigated the use of a replication-deficient herpes simplex viral (HSV) vector with the human TNFα gene in a sarcoma-bearing rat model and found that ILuP produced lung levels of TNFα that decreased tumor growth significantly, but not significantly different than those achieved by ILuP with HSV amplicons without the TNFα gene [40]. When the weakly immunogenic CC531S carcinoma tumor was injected in WAG/Rij rats and perfusion with recombinant human TNFα was performed, no significant anti-tumor responses were seen [34]. Similar poor results were also seen in experiments of isolated limb perfusion when non-immunogenic BN 175 sarcoma-bearing rats were perfused with recombinant human TNFα in a well-oxygenated isolated limb perfusion setting. However, short ischemic anoxia resulted in impressive tumor response characteristic for TNFα [41].

Significant toxicities have been seen in several clinical trials after even small intravenous doses of TNFα administration, especially hypotension, inflammation at the site of injection, thrombocytopenia, and neurologic symptoms. [42]. Therefore, it has been of utmost importance to test the feasibility of ILuP with TNFα in pig studies. Pogrebniak and colleagues treated eight animals with left-sided ILuP with TNFα in a dose up to 80 μg/kg, and three animals with 40 μg/kg at moderate hyperthermia (39°C) for 60 to 90 minutes [22]. None of the pigs treated with 80 μg/kg survived the procedure, probably because of the high systemic TNFα levels that were seen (up to 340 ± 220 ng/mL). Systemic leakage was also seen in pigs perfused with lower doses of TNFα but the procedure was better-tolerated, with the mean arterial pressure being only minimally affected by an elevated pulmonary artery pressure and decreased cardiac output. Pigs that underwent hyperthermic ILuP demonstrated acute subpleural and peribronchial edema along with neutrophilic infiltration, whereas one pig needed a pneumonectomy to survive the procedure. Although no clinically evident long-term sequelae were seen in surviving pigs, this study clearly demonstrates that leakage control is of utmost importance when ILuP with TNFα is considered, because complete absolute isolation of the lung is not possible. Therefore, continuous measurement of systemic levels caused by leakage are absolutely indicated when performing ILuP studies with TNFα.

In 1996, Pass and colleagues reported the results of a phase I trial of ILuP with TNFα in 15 patients (16 procedures) with lung metastases from sarcoma, melanoma, renal cell, colorectal, and adenoid cystic carcinoma [13]. A complete metastasectomy was performed in only three patients, and one patient with bilateral lung metastases had a staged bilateral lung perfusion. Doses of 0.3 mg, 0.6 mg, 1 mg, 3 mg, and 6.0 mg of TNFα were tested, combined with a fixed dose of interferon-γ. Excellent isolation was obtained as demonstrated by online immunoassay. However, one patient demonstrated systemic leakage of 10% of the dose delivered to the lung. This patient required re-intubation and vasopressor support for pulmonary insufficiency with bilateral infiltrates and bronchorrhea, probably because of high TNFα levels but probably amplified by hyperthermic treatment of the lung to 45°C. A maximum tolerated dose (MTD) of 6 mg of TNFα was found in this study.

Cisplatin/carboplatin

Rat and pig models, and one human phase I trial with cisplatin (CDDP) or its derivative, carboplatin, have been reported since 1994 by different groups. ILuP with CDDP was tested by Ellis and colleagues [43] and by Li and colleagues [44] in a rat model of sarcoma lung metastases, and of carcinoma lung metastases by Van Putte and colleagues [45]. Ellis performed ILuP in a bilateral pulmonary metastases model and showed significant tumor reduction in the perfused left lung as compared with the right untreated lung or intravenous therapy [43]. The lung levels of CDDP were significantly higher after ILuP compared with intravenous therapy, whereas systemic exposure was less as expressed by platelet count. Li and colleagues described a model of a solitary tumor nodule by injection of sarcoma cells directly into the lung parenchyma instead of intravenous injection [44]. Rats underwent ILuP with 0.1, 0.25, and 0.5 mg/mL of CDDP, and only 0.1 mg/mL was well-tolerated and used for efficacy studies. These experiments showed much higher CDDP concentra-

tion in the tumor compared with intravenous injection with lower systemic exposure. Tumor weight 3 weeks after treatment was significantly lower after ILuP compared with controls or intravenously treated rats. CDDP concentration in the perfused lung tissue was dependent on both the perfusate CDDP concentration and ILuP time [46,47]. However, CDDP concentration in the tumor tissue was related to tumor weight as soon as the perfusate concentration of CDDP exceeded 25 μg/mL, with smaller tumors demonstrating higher levels [47]. Both the antitumor effect and tumor levels of CDDP increased when the MTD of 20 μmol/L of digitonin was added [48]. The additive effect of digitonin is explained by the increased intracellular uptake of cisplatin by increasing the permeability of the plasma membrane by binding of digitonin to cholesterol [49,50]. Ratto and colleagues tested a higher doses of CDDP (2.5 mg/kg and 5 mg/kg in piglets of 30 to 35 kg for a respective level of 0.15 mg/mL and 0.30 mg/mL), and compared a 1-hour lung infusion through the pulmonary artery without venous control with ILuP. Higher CDDP lung levels and lower systemic exposure were seen after ILuP that with the regional infusion, whereas similar acute histologic (but reversible) changes were seen for 2.5 and 5 mg/kg of CDDP [51]. ILuP with CDDP has also been studied in a pig model at dose of 150 mg/m^2 and 300 mg/m^2 with normothermia, and 300mg/m^2 of CDDP at 41.5°C [52], with these groups being compared with control animals and a sham group. After 40 minutes of left ILuP, the right lung was removed and lung function parameters were observed for 6 hours, after which biopsy samples were taken for histologic quantification of acute lung injury. None of the pigs died during reperfusion of the left lung and no statistical significant differences in hemodynamic, ventilatory, and gas exchange parameters were seen between perfusion groups. However, histological damage was more frequently seen in the group with 300 mg/m^2 compared with all other groups, although the damage was less when hyperthermia was added. A correlation between CDDP perfusion concentration and CDDP lung tissue levels was demonstrated, although the highest levels for the group of 300 mg/m^2 (±70 μg/gm tissue) seemed lower compared with the study by Ratto (±100 μg/gm tissue). Ratto had performed a feasibility trial of ILuP with a fixed dose of 200 mg/m^2 of CDDP, comparable to the 5 mg/kg of his piglets study, and published the results of these six patients in 1996 [14]. Four patients had unilateral ILuP, whereas in two patients staged bilateral perfusions were performed. Sarcoma metastases were treated by ILuP for 60 minutes at normothermia, followed by a complete metastasectomy, but without control over the bronchial circulation. All patients survived the procedure but pulmonary edema occurred after 48 hours in two patients, necessitating respiratory support in one for 5 days. No difference between lung and tumor CDDP levels were observed, although they were very high at 70 µg/gm of tissue. Lung function tests 90 days after the perfusion demonstrated a significant decrease in all parameters but arterial pO_2 and pCO_2. Pulmonary function was reassessed in only two patients after 12 months, and these showed improvement over postoperative values, although they were still below preoperative values. Two other clinical studies described ILuP with CDDP. The first study was reported by Johnston and colleagues [7] as part of a feasibility trial in which doxorubicin was also tested. Two patients were treated with 14 to 20 µg/mL of CDDP (dose in mg/m^2 was not given) and excellent separation of the systemic and pulmonary circulations were demonstrated. A second study was reported by Schröder and colleagues [53], who used ILuP with 70 mg/m^2 of CDDP and hyperthermia (41°C) in four patients after complete metastasectomy. No systemic drug-related toxicity was seen, although all four patients experienced transient pulmonary toxicity grade 1 to 2, which resolved within 12 weeks. Recently, a video-assisted technique of ILuP (VATS-ILuP) in dogs has been developed [20]. This technique combined endovascular placement of a Swan-Ganz catheter into the pulmonary artery with thoracoscopic placement of two venous cannulae connected to a suction device. A single-pass system was used and ILuP performed for 20 minutes at a flow rate of 30 mL/min with 50 µg/mL of CDDP. VATS-ILuP in five dogs was compared with conventional single-pass ILuP in five dogs, and no differences between groups were seen except for a smaller incision and better weight recovery in the VATS-ILuP group.

Doxorubicin

Doxorubicin is an anthracycline antibiotic with proven clinical activity against a number of malignancies such as breast, bile duct, endometrial, esophageal, and liver carcinoma, as well as non-Hodgkin lymphoma, soft tissue, and osteosarcoma [54]. Because of its efficacy in treating sarcoma, and because systemic administration of high-dose doxorubicin results in congestive heart failure caused by degenerative cardiomyopathy, doxorubicin has been frequently explored for locoregional application.

The first ILuP experiments with doxorubicin were performed by Minchin and Boyd in an ex vivo rat model [55] and by Johnston in dogs [5]. Minchin

found a linear relation between increasing perfusate doxorubicin concentration and lung concentration without a plateau phase. These results were not seen in the lungs of dogs, suggesting a difference in doxorubicin uptake between species [56]. The plateau phase was seen in dogs after 40 minutes, and increasing the perfusate concentration did not increase lung tissue levels more than 125 nmol/g (72.5 µg/mL). Johnson and colleagues performed a feasibility trial to determine the optimal perfusion technique by perfusing 5 dogs with a concentration of 0.5 µg/mL. The perfusate was hypothermic (23–25°C) and whole blood (hematocrit 40%) in an attempt to protect the lungs and reduce lung edema. These experiments showed a high degree of isolation of the lung with no detectable systemic leakage and a perfusate concentration more than 0.2 µg/mL during 45 minutes [5]. This is significantly higher than achieved by systemic therapy, during which plasma concentrations of patients receiving 40 to 60 mg/m^2 decreased to 0.05 µg/mL after 60 minutes [57]. Irreversible lung damage was seen with lung tissue levels between 10 and 20 µg/gm [5]. Histologic damage was seen in dogs after hyperthermic IluP (39°C) used by Baciewicz and colleagues, with tissue levels of 20.6±4.5 µg/g and perfusate concentrations more than 7.61 µg/mL [9]. At lower temperatures, tissue damage was seen with perfusate concentrations of 11.6 µg/mL [8]. All but one dog survived left ILuP with subsequent right pneumonectomy in the study by Baciewicz, even though lung tissue levels were higher than in the experiments by Johnston [5]. The differences in perfusate and lung levels achieved and differences in survival may be attributed to the difference in perfusate temperature (39°C) and the lower hematocrit (20%).

Toxicity experiments in Fisher rats by the Memorial Sloan-Kettering group found a MTD of 320 µg/mL of doxorubcin (±5.1 mg/kg) [32], whereas the LD$_{50}$ of rats after 2 months for doxorubicin was determined to be a perfusate concentration of 10 µg/mL [15]. Efficacy experiments showed significant tumor reduction in the left treated lung of sarcoma-bearing rats with 320 µg/mL of doxorubicin, and the perfused left lung was disease-free macroscopically in 90% and disease-free microscopically in 30% [32]. In a subsequent study by Ng and colleagues in which ILuP with 320 µg/mL of doxorubicin was compared with intravenous therapy, a MTD of perfused doxorubicin of 7 mg/kg was determined as reflected by reduction in weight, cardiac output, and hematologic toxicity. The intravenously treated rats experienced significantly greater morbidity, including severe hematologic toxicity (decreased haemoglobin), decreased cardiac index (30% reduction), and failure to gain weight [58], and

ILuP achieved significantly higher lung levels than systemic therapy [59]. The problem of development of tumor resistance to cytostatic agents and radiation therapy was studied by Port in 1995 [60]. He pretreated rats with buthionine sulfoximine, a potent inhibitor of glutathione synthesis, after which ILuP with doxorubicin at 10 μg/mL was administered. Compared with intravenously treated rats (who had more than 500 nodules), significantly fewer tumor nodules (16±22) were seen after ILuP [60]. Long-term survival after ILuP with doxorubicin was further evaluated in a unilateral lung metastasis model. Rats treated with left ILuP with 6.4 mg/kg (~320 μg/mL) of doxorubicin had a median survival time of 36 days, which was significantly longer compared with control animals (20 days), and two ILuP rats were found to be disease-free after 6 weeks [36].

So far, the feasibility studies by Minchin and colleagues [56] in three patients and by Johnston and colleagues [7] in six patients have been followed by two phase I studies [15,61]. Both of these studies explored the toxicity of doxorubicin at normothermia in patients who experienced unresectable sarcomatous pulmonary metastases. Burt and colleagues perfused eight patients during 20 minutes with a flow of 300 to 500 mL/min, administering doses between 40 and 80 mg/m². Substantial lung damage was seen at more than 40 mg/m². Lung tissue levels varied from 1.3 to 57.3 μg/g [15], and the maximum perfusate concentration was determined to be 12.9 μg/mL. An unpublished study by Putnam described 16 patients who underwent ILuP with doses of doxorubicin between 60 to 75 mg/m² during 30 minutes. An operative mortality of 18.8% was seen, whereas lung levels varied between 74 and 2750 μg/g [61].

Melphalan

Melphalan (MN) is one of the alkylating agents, which are a group of drugs that are effective against many types of malignancy, with their use being limited by hematopoietic toxicity. Since 1996, ILuP with MN has been tested in models of metastatic carcinoma [34] and sarcoma [62] to the lung. Toxicity studies attempted to determine the MTD of MN, whereas acute [34,62] and long-term [63,64] efficacy was evaluated in tumor-bearing rats. MTD of 8 mg/kg of MN was initially found, but in a subsequent study early survival rates after left ILuP and contralateral right pneumonectomy were less for animals treated with the dose of 8 mg/kg than with lower doses and a MTD of 4 mg/kg was used for further studies. In

addition, MN was combined with TNFα because of the excellent results seen with isolated limb perfusion [4], and doses up to 8 mg/kg of MN with 800 μg/kg of TNFα were found to be tolerable [34]. All rats that received 4 mg/kg of MN intravenously survived, whereas after treatment with 8 mg/kg, a 100% mortality rate was seen by 5 days. Histologic analysis of the perfused left lung showed limited areas of alveolar exudation, alveolar cell hyperplasia, and varying degrees of pleural fibrosis and pleuritis for doses up to 8 mg/kg [34].

The number of carcinoma and sarcoma tumors in the treated lung was significantly less in animals receiving MN via IluP than in animals receiving MN intravenously. In addition, MN ILuP resulted in a significant reduction of tumor nodules in the IluP-treated left lung as compared with the contralateral and untreated right lung [34,62]. Also, survival was significantly better in the ILuP group than in intravenously treated rats [63,64]. No signs of progressive toxicity in the IluP-treated lung were observed during an observation period up to 6 months [63,64]. ILuP with combination therapy of MN with TNFα, cisplatin, or gemcitabine was also tested by our group [34,45]. Although no benefit was seen with the addition of TNFα and cisplatin when compared with monotherapy with MN, a clear synergistic effect was demonstrated when ILuP with MN was combined with increasing doses of gemcitabine in vitro, resulting in significantly longer survival.

Many pharmacokinetic studies have been performed since 1996 with MN. These studies showed that lung levels of MN were up to 50-times higher after ILuP than after intravenous treatment. When MN was measured in the pulmonary venous effluent of ILuP-treated rats, MN levels increased maximally within 2 minutes and remained almost constant throughout perfusion for all doses (2 mg/kg to 8 mg/kg). Five minutes after washout, MN levels of the venous effluent decreased to zero, and during or after ILuP no MN was detected in the systemic serum. These studies demonstrated excellent absorption by lung tissue and a good first-pass effect [34,62]. Further pharmacokinetic experiments demonstrated that lung and tumor levels of MN were not significantly different between ILuP with 0.5 mg of MN delivered with a single-pass technique compared with a closed loop recirculating circuit [27]. Therefore, it makes no difference in final MN lung and tumor levels whether a fixed MN concentration is given to the lung tissue or a bolus of MN is injected into the circuit. Although the total MN lung levels are not affected by changes in perfusion flow, MN concentration, or duration of perfusion, it has been demonstrated that such alterations will lead to differing MN levels in different parts of the lung [65,66]. When MN delivered to the lung with the standard technique of anterograde IluP was compared with retrograde IluP, lung levels were higher for the apex and the base of the lung, but lower in the hilum and not significantly different in the periphery of the lung [66].

In 2004, our group reported on the results of a phase I trial of ILuP with MN for patients with resectable lung metastases [16]. Between 2001 and 2003, 16 patients had 21 procedures for a variety of tumors, like colorectal carcinoma, renal cell carcinoma, sarcoma, and salivary gland tumors. Patients with bilateral lung metastases underwent staged thoracotomies with an interval of 4 to 8 weeks between to allow for the observation of delayed toxicity. ILuP was performed for 30 minutes with MN after a stabilization period for flow, leakage, and temperature. The 30-minute perfusion time was chosen because pharmacokinetic studies of MN effluens levels demonstrated no advantage for longer perfusion procedures with MN [67], because reperfusion after prolonged pulmonary ischemia during ILuP results in significant inflammatory changes [68] and addition of a membrane oxygenator can act as a filter for the MN in the circuit. At the end of ILuP and washout, a complete metastasectomy including hilar and mediastinal lymphadenectomy was performed. Two temperature levels (37°C and 42°C) were tested for each dose level. The levels of 15, 30, and 45 mg were well-tolerated but dose-limiting toxicity was seen at the level of 60 mg at 37°C (Fig. 8). Therefore,

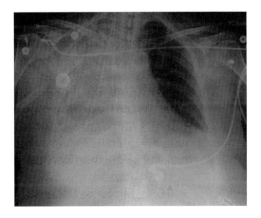

Fig. 8. Chemical pneumonitis at day 2 after isolated lung perfusion at the right side in patient 19 (level 7). (*From* Hendriks JM, Grootenboers MJ, Schramel FM, et al. Isolated lung perfusion with melphalan for respectable lung metastases: a phase I clinical trial. Ann Thorac Surg 2004; 78:1919–27; with permission.)

the MTD of ILuP with MN was 45 mg at 42°C [16]. To obtain more meaningful pharmacokinetic data, this phase I trial was expanded for the dose levels of 15 mg and 45 mg up to 10 patients and toxicity was also recorded. This extension study showed significantly more toxicity for the hyperthermia level compared with normothermia, whereas lung levels were not significantly different (unpublished data).

Gemcitabine

$2',2'$-Difluorodeoxycytidine (dFdC, gemcitabine) is a nucleoside analog of deoxycytidine with clinical activity against ovarian, breast, pancreas, colorectal, and non-small cell lung carcinoma (NSCLC) [69,70]. In vitro studies with gemcitabine (GCB) showed cell kill that is concentration- and time-dependent, which is the main argument for local regional anticancer therapy [71]. The MTD in rats has been evaluated either after ILuP or intravenous therapy using a dose-escalating schedule from 20 up to 320 mg/kg. The MTD by systemic treatment was 160 mg/kg, whereas the MTD by left ILuP was 320 mg/kg. No severe histologic damage was seen after a period of 90 days. [72]. Significant higher lung tissue levels were found after ILuP than after intravenous therapy [71]. Lung tissue was already saturated after 6 minutes of ILuP and continued treatment to 30 minutes led to significantly worse pulmonary edema. Delayed restoration of the circulation to 60 minutes after ILuP rather than immediate restoration after decannulation led to significantly higher lung levels (+456% at 30 minutes, and +828% at 60 minutes) (Van Putte, unpublished data). Efficacy studies of ILuP with GCB in the unilateral model of pulmonary metastatic colorectal adenocarcinoma demonstrated a significantly longer survival for ILuP-treated rats (320 mg/kg) compared with untreated control animals and intravenously treated rats (160 mg/kg) (Van Putte, unpublished data). Because the basis of anticancer treatment consists of systemic administration of a combination of several chemotherapeutics to interfere with several target mechanisms [73], combining several drugs together with different cytostatic targets may result in synergistic actions. Therefore, ILuP with combinations of GCB, CDDP, and MN was evaluated both in vitro by using sulforhodamine B (SRB) cell assay and in vivo using the unilateral metastatic pulmonary adenocarcinoma model in the rat [45]. In vitro, CC531s adenocarcinoma cells were incubated with a single agent (CDDP, MN, or GCB) or with a combination of two drugs. One drug was added at a concentration causing 25% growth inhibition (IC25), whereas the other drug was added at variable concentrations. Synergistic activity was observed for the combination of GCB and MN, whereas other combinations showed only an additive or antagonistic activity. In vivo, different groups of rats had single-agent ILuP with GCB, MN, and CDDP, whereas three more groups had ILuP using combinations of two agents. Survival until death caused by metastatic disease was compared with untreated control rats. Single-agent therapy with all tested drugs resulted in significantly longer survival compared with untreated controls, whereas synergistic action was seen after ILuP with the combination of GCB and MN compared with all groups, and the combination of MN and CDDP compared with single-agent ILuP with CDDP or MN. No animals survived to the end of the 90-day follow-up period except for rats that were treated with the combination of GCB and MN (67% survival).

Paclitaxel

The use of paclitaxel as a prototypic taxane for regional lung delivery was investigated by Schrump and colleagues [23]. The drug was selected over other taxanes because of its broad spectrum of activity against solid tumors and minimal pulmonary toxicity at doses up to 700 mg/m^2 over 24 hours [74]. The dose-limiting toxicity in humans after intravenous therapy has been neurologic and occurred at doses more than the MTD of 225 mg/m^2 (15 μmol/L) [75]. In a sheep model, Schrump and colleagues [23] administered paclitaxel by retrograde hyperthermia ILuP for 90 minutes with the use of a membrane oxygenator [23]. A dose escalation starting at 20 mg and progressing up to 800 mg (320 μmol/L) was performed. This did not show a plateau phase at the highest dose and no pulmonary toxicity was observed within 3 hours after ILuP. Systemic plasma concentrations after ILuP with the MTD were far below the levels seen after intravenous therapy, showing that paclitaxel is not rapidly released from the lung after ILuP. Paclitaxel has also been shown to be effective in vitro against several cancer cell lines with enhanced toxicity by achieved by hyperthermia for both epithelial lines, as well as paclitaxel-resistant cell lines such as sarcoma and melanoma.

FUDR

Standard intravenous regimens for stage III (Dukes C) colon cancer include combinations of fluorouracil-based regimens with new drugs, like oxaliplatin [76]. The fluorinated pyrimidines, like FUDR and 5-FU, have been among the most active agents in the treatment of colorectal adenocarcinoma for more than 45 years, but their systemic use is limited by extensive myelosuppression and gastrointestinal distress. FUDR (2′-deoxy-5-fluorouridine) was tested in 1995 as a single agent for ILuP in BDIX rats with K12/TRb colon adenocarcinoma lung metastases [33]. These experiments showed a significant reduction of both the number and size of tumor nodules in the ILuP-treated left lung compared with the untreated right lung, untreated animals, or intravenously treated rats [33]. The drug could be administered in a dose as high as 840 mg/kg, far above the LD50 after in-

Table 2
Human ILuP studies

Year	Author	Ref.	Drug	Lung temperature (°C)	N of patients	Perfusion time (min)	Operable	MTD
1958	Creech	3	Mitomycin C + nitrogen mustard + 5FU	NA	21	NA	Yes	NA
1984	Minchin	56	Doxorubicin	25	3	50	No	NA
1995	Johnston	7	Doxorubicin/ Cisplatin	NA	8	45–60	No	NA
1996	Pass	13	TNF-α	38–39.5	19	90	No	6 mg
1996	Ratto	14	Cisplatin	37	6	60	Yes	200 mg/m^2 (fixed)
2000	Burt	15	Doxorubicin	37	8	20	No	40 mg/m^2
2000	Putnam	61	Doxorubicin	37	16	NA	No	60 mg/m^2
2002	Schröder	53	Cisplatin	41	4	21–40	Both	70 mg/m^2 (fixed)
2004	Hendriks	16	Melphalan	37–42	16 (21 procedures)	30	Yes	45 mg – 42°C

Abbreviation: NA, not available.

travenous therapy of 670 mg/kg [77]. These findings make FUDR an interesting agent for ILuP, either as a single agent or in combined regimens.

Prospects

Since 1983, the number of scientific publications addressing ILuP has rapidly increased Many models have been developed to test both chemotherapeutic and biological agents for efficacy and pharmacokinetic profile, which have largely proven to be superior to systemic therapy. The technique proved to be safe in humans, and phase I trials in humans have been completed for most of the drugs tested in animal models [13–16,61] (Table 2). Phase II and III trials are needed to test the efficacy of combined metastasectomy with ILuP for improving local recurrence rates and survival. It is our opinion that successful completion of such studies will require the cooperation of multiple centers. Task forces are needed to standardize ILuP for drugs, flow rates, perfusate composition, temperature, and many other parameters. New drugs will soon be tested, as well as novel combinations to optimize the effectiveness of a single ILuP treatment, as demonstrated by Van Putte and colleagues [45]. Regional lung perfusion with inflow occlusion (Fig. 9) is inferior to ILuP pharmacokinetically but superior to the intravenous adminstration of nitrogen mustard [78], doxorubicin [79–81], cisplatin [51], and gemcitabine [72]. More studies are needed to explore regional lung perfusion techniques as neoadjuvant or adjuvant therapy with metastasectomy and ILuP. In addition, regional lung therapy can also become a valuable tool for local gene therapy [40,82].

A   **B**

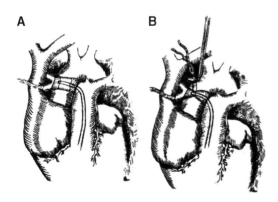

Fig. 9. Methods used to occlude the pulmonary artery. (*A*) Balloon-tipped double lumen cardiac catheter. (*B*) Single lumen cardiac catheter with a snare around the pulmonary artery. (*From* Smyth N, Blades B. Selective chemotherapy of the lung during unilateral pulmonary artery occlusion with a balloon-tipped catheter. J Thorac Cardiovasc Surg 1960; 40:653–66; with permission.)

References

[1] Ranney D. Drug targeting to the lungs. Biochem Pharmacol 1986;35:1063–9.

[2] Pastorino U, Buyse M, Friedel G, et al. Long-term results of lung metastasectomy: prognostic analyses based on 5206 cases. The International Registry of Lung Metastases. J Thorac Cardiovasc Surg 1997;113: 37–49.

[3] Creech O, Krementz ET, Ryan RF, et al. Chemotherapy of cancer: regional perfusion utilizing an extracorporeal circuit. Ann Surg 1958;148:616–32.

[4] Eggermont A, de Wilt J, ten Hagen T. Current uses of isolated limb perfusion in the clinic and a model system for new strategies. Review Article. Lancet Oncol 2003;4:429–37.

[5] Johnston MR, Minchin R, Shull JH, et al. Isolated lung perfusion with adriamycin. A preclinical study. Cancer 1983;52:404–9.

[6] Johnston MR, Christensen CW, Minchin RF, et al. Isolated total lung perfusion as a means to deliver organ-specific chemotherapy: long-term studies in animals. Surgery 1985;98:35–44.

[7] Johnston MR, Minchen RF, Dawson CA. Lung perfusion with chemotherapy in patients with unresectable metastatic sarcoma to the lung or diffuse bronchioloalveolar carcinoma. J Thorac Cardiovasc Surg 1995; 110:368–73.

[8] Minchin RF, Johnston MR, Schuller HM, et al. Pulmonary toxicity of doxorubicin administered by in situ isolated lung perfusion in dogs. Cancer 1988;61: 1320–5.

[9] Baciewicz FA, Arredondo M, Chaudhuri B, et al. Pharmacokinetics and toxicity of isolated lung perfusion of lung with doxorubicin. J Surg Res 1991;50:124–8.

[10] Bongard R, Roerig D, Johnston M, et al. Influence of temperature and plasma protein on doxorubicin uptake by isolated lungs. Drug Metab Dispos 1993;21: 428–34.

[11] Rickaby D, Fehring J, Johnston M, et al. Tolerance of the isolated perfused lung to hyperthermia. J Thorac Cardiovasc Surg 1991;101:732–9.

[12] Cowen M, Mulvin D, Howard R, et al. Lung tolerance to hyperthermia by in vivo perfusion. Eur J Cardio-thorac Surg 1992;6:167–73.

[13] Pass HI, Mew DJ, Kranda KC, et al. Isolated lung perfusion with tumor necrosis factor for pulmonary metastases. Ann Thorac Surg 1996;61:1609–17.

[14] Ratto GB, Toma S, Civalleri D, et al. Isolated lung perfusion with platinum in the treatment of pulmonary metastases from soft tissue sarcomas. J Thorac Cardiovasc Surg 1996;112:614–22.

[15] Burt ME, Liu D, Abolhoda A, et al. Isolated lung perfusion for patients with unresectable metastases from

sarcoma: a phase I trial. Ann Thorac Surg 2000;69: 1542–9.

[16] Hendriks JM, Grootenboers MJ, Schramel FM, et al. Isolated lung perfusion with melphalan for resectable lung metastases: a phase I clinical trial. Ann Thorac Surg 2004;78:1919–27.

[17] Miller B, Rosenbaum A. The vascular supply to metastatic tumors of the lung. Surg Gynecol Obstet 1967; 125:1009–16.

[18] Milne E, Noonan C, Margulis A, et al. Vascular supply of pulmonary metastases. Experimental study in rats. Invest Radiol 1969;4:215–29.

[19] Haller J, Bron K, Wholey M, et al. Selective bronchial artery catheterization for diagnostic and physiologic studies and chemotherapy for bronchogenic carcinoma. J Thorac Cardiovasc Surg 1966;51:143–52.

[20] Jinbo M, Ueda K, Kaneda Y, et al. Video-assisted transcatheter lung perfusion regional chemotherapy. Eur J Cardiothorac Surg 2005;27:1079–82.

[21] Furrer M, Lardinois D, Thormann W, et al. Isolated lung perfusion: single-pass system versus recirculating blood perfusion in pigs. Ann Thorac Surg 1998;65: 1420–5.

[22] Pogrebniak H, Witt C, Terrill R, et al. Isolated lung perfusion with tumor necrosis factor: a swine model in preparation of human trials. Ann Thorac Surg 1994; 57:1477–83.

[23] Schrump DS, Zhai S, Nguyen DM, et al. Pharmacokinetics of paclitaxel administered by hyperthermic retrograde isolated lung perfusion techniques. J Thorac Cardiovasc Surg 2002;123:686–94.

[24] Weksler B, Schneider A, Ng B, et al. Isolated single lung perfusion in the rat. J Appl Physiol 1993;74: 2736–9.

[25] Wang HY, Port JL, Hochwald S, et al. Revised technique of isolated lung perfusion in the rat. Ann Thorac Surg 1995;60:211–2.

[26] Hendriks J, Van Schil P, Eyskens E. Modified technique of isolated left lung perfusion in the rat. Eur Surg Res 1999;31:93–6.

[27] Van Putte BP, Hendriks JMH, Romijn S, et al. Single-pass isolated lung perfusion versus recirculating isolated lung perfusion with melphalan in a rat model. Ann Thorac Surg 2002;74:893–8.

[28] Krueger T, Kümmerie A, Vallet C, et al. Antegrade and retrograde isolated lung perfusion with doxorubicin in the rat: comparison of pharmacokinetics and toxicity. Eur Respir J 2002;20:s179.

[29] Romijn S, Hendriks J, Van Putte B, et al. Anterograde versus retrograde isolated lung perfusion with melphalan in the WAG-Rij rat. Eur J Cardiothorac Surg 2005; 27:1083–5.

[30] Nawata S, Abolhoda A, Ross H, et al. Sequential bilateral isolated lung perfusion in the rat: an experimental model. Ann Thorac Surg 1997;63:796–9.

[31] Blades B, Pierpoint H, Samadi A, et al. Effect of experimental lung ischemia on pulmonary function: a preliminary report. Surg Forum 1953;4:255.

[32] Weksler B, Lenert J, Ng B, et al. Isolated single lung perfusion with doxorubicin is effective in eradicating soft tissue sarcoma lung metastases in a rat model. J Thorac Cardiovasc Surg 1994;107:50–4.

[33] Ng B, Lenert JT, Weksler B, et al. Isolated lung perfusion with FUDR is an effective treatment for colorectal adenocarcinoma lung metastases in rats. Ann Thorac Surg 1995;59:205–8.

[34] Hendriks JM, Van Schil PE, De Boeck G, et al. Isolated lung perfusion with melphalan and tumor necrosis factor for metastatic pulmonary adenocarcinoma. Ann Thorac Surg 1998;66:1719–25.

[35] Wexler H. Accurate identification of experimental pulmonary metastases. J Natl Cancer Instit 1966;36: 641–5.

[36] Abolhoda A, Brooks A, Nawata S, et al. Isolated lung perfusion with doxorubicin prolongs survival in a rodent model of pulmonary metastases. Ann Thorac Surg 1997;64:181–4.

[37] Linder A, Friedel G, Fritz P, et al. The ex-vivo isolated, perfused human lung model: description and potential applications. Thorac Cardiovasc Surg 1996; 44:140–6.

[38] Asher A, Mulé JJ, Reichert C, et al. Studies on the antitumor efficacy of systemically administered recombinant tumor necrosis factor against several murine tumors in vivo. J Immunol 1987;138:963–74.

[39] Weksler B, Blumberg D, Lenert J, et al. Isolated single-lung perfusion with TNF-α in a rat sarcoma lung metastases model. Ann Thorac Surg 1994;58: 328–32.

[40] Brooks A, Ng B, Liu D, et al. Specific organ gene transfer in vivo by regional organ perfusion with herpes viral amplicon vectors: implications for local gene therapy. Surgery 2001;129:324–34.

[41] Manusama E, Durante N, Marquet R, et al. Ischemia promotes anti-tumor effect of tumour necrosis factor alpha in isolated limb perfusion in the rat. Reg Cancer Treat 1994;7:155–9.

[42] Fraker DL, Alexander HR, Pass HI. Biologic therapy of tumor necrosis factor: clinical applications by systemic and regional administration. In: DeVita V, Hellman S, Rosenberg SA, editors. Biologic therapy of cancer. 2nd ed. Philadelphia: Lippincott; 1995. p. 329–46.

[43] Ellis J, Ng B, Port J, et al. Isolated lung perfusion with carboplatin for metastatic sarcoma in the F344 rat. Surg Forum 1994; XLV:294–5.

[44] Li TS, Sugi K, Ueda K, et al. Isolated lung perfusion with cisplatin in a rat lung solitary tumor nodule model. Anticancer Res 1998;18:4171–6.

[45] Van Putte BP, Hendriks JM, Romijn S, et al. Combination chemotherapy with gemcitabine with isolated lung perfusion for the treatment of pulmonary metastases. J Thorac Cardiovasc Surg 2005;130: 125–30.

[46] Li TS, Kaneda Y, Saeki K, et al. Pharmacokinetic differences between rat tumour and lung tissues following isolated lung perfusion with cisplatin. Eur J Cancer 1999;35:1846–50.

[47] Saeki K, Kaneda Y, Li TS, et al. Pharmacokinetic characteristic in tumor tissue following isolated lung perfusion with CDDP – an experimental study in solitary pulmonary sarcoma model in rat. J Surg Oncol 2000; 75:193–6.

[48] Tanaka T, Kaneda Y, Li TS, et al. Digitonin enhances the antitumor effect of cisplatin during isolated lung perfusion. Ann Thorac Surg 2001;72:1173–8.

[49] Miller R. Interaction between digitonin and bilayer membranes. Biochim Biophys Acta 1984;774:151–7.

[50] Vercesi A, Bernardes C, Hoffmann M, et al. Digitonin permeabilization doest not affect mitochondrial function and allows the determination of the mitochondrial membrane potential of Trypansosoma cruzi in situ. J Biol Chem 1991;266:14431–4.

[51] Ratto G, Esposito M, Leprini A, et al. In situ lung perfusion with cisplatin. Cancer 1993;71:2962–70.

[52] Franke U, Wittwer H, Kaluza M, et al. Evaluation of isolated lung perfusion as neoadjuvant therapy of lung metastases using a novel in vivo pig model: II. High-dose cisplatin is well tolerated by the native lung tissue. Eur J Cardiothorac Surg 2004;26:800–6.

[53] Schröder C, Fisher S, Pieck AC, et al. Technique and results of hyperthermic isolated lung perfusion with high-doses of cisplatin for the treatment of surgically relapsing or unresectable lung sarcoma metastasis. Eur J Cardiothorac Surg 2002;22: 41–6.

[54] Gewirtz DA. A critical evaluation of the mechanisms of action proposed for the antitumor effects of the anthracycline antibiotics adriamycin and daunorubicin. Biochem Pharmacol 1999;57:727–41.

[55] Minchin RF, Boyd MR. Uptake and metabolism of doxorubicin in isolated perfused rat lung. Biochem Pharmacol 1983;32:2829–32.

[56] Minchin RF, Johnston MR, Aiken MA, et al. Pharmacokinetics of doxorubicin in isolated lung of dogs and humans perfused in vivo. J Pharmacol Exp Ther 1984; 229:193–8.

[57] Benjamin R, Riggs C, Bachur N. Plasma pharmacokinetics of adriamycin and its metabolites in humans with normal hepatic and renal function. Cancer Res 1977;37:1416–20.

[58] Ng B, Hochwald S, Burt M. Isolated lung perfusion with doxorubicin reduces cardiac and host toxicities associated with systemic administration. Ann Thorac Surg 1996;61:969–72.

[59] Weksler B, Ng B, Lenert J, et al. Isolated single-lung perfusion with doxorubicin is pharmacokinetically superior to intravenous injection. Ann Thorac Surg 1993; 56:209–14.

[60] Port J, Hochwald S, Wang H, et al. Buthionine sufoximine pre-treatment potentiates the effect of isolated lung perfusion with doxorubicin. Ann Thorac Surg 1995;60:239–43.

[61] Putnam Jr JB. New and evolving treatment methods for pulmonary metastases. Semin Thorac Cardiovasc Surg 2002;14:49–56.

[62] Nawata S, Abecasis N, Ross H, et al. Isolated lung perfusion with melphalan for the treatment of metastatic pulmonary sarcoma. J Thorac Cardiovasc Surg 1996;112:1542–8.

[63] Ueda K, Sugi K, Li TS, et al. The long-term evaluation of pulmonary toxicity following isolated lung perfusion with melphalan in the rat. Anticancer Res 1999; 19:141–8.

[64] Hendriks JM, Van Schil PE, Van Oosterom AA, et al. Isolated lung perfusion with melphalan prolongs survival in a rat model of metastatic pulmonary adenocarcinoma. Eur Surg Res 1999;31:267–71.

[65] Romijn S, Hendriks J, Van Putte B, et al. Variations in flow, duration and concentration do not change the final lung concentration of melphalan after isolated lung perfusion in rats. Eur Surg Res 2003;35: 50–3.

[66] Romijn S, Hendriks J, Van Putte B, et al. Regional differences of melphalan lung levels after isolated lung perfusion in the rat. J Surg Res 2005;125: 157–60.

[67] Briele H, Djuric M, Jung D, et al. Pharmacokinetics of melphalan in clinical isolated perfusion of the extremities. Cancer Res 1985;45:1885–9.

[68] Abolhoda A, Brooks A, Choudhry M, et al. Characterization of local inflammatory response in an isolated lung perfusion model. Ann Surg Oncol 1998;5:87–92.

[69] Sandler A, Ettinger DS. Gemcitabine: single-agent and combination therapy in non-small cell lung cancer. Oncologist 1999;4:241–51.

[70] Storniolo AM, Enas NH, Brown CA, et al. An investigational new drug treatment program for patients with gemcitabine: results for over 3000 patients with pancreatic carcinoma. Cancer (Phila.) 1999;85:1261–8.

[71] Van Putte BP, Hendriks JM, Romijn S, et al. Isolated lung perfusion with gemcitabine in a rat: pharmacokinetics and survival. J Surg Res 2003;109:118–22.

[72] Van Putte BP, Hendriks JM, Romijn S, et al. Pharmacokinetics after pulmonary artery perfusion with gemcitabine. Ann Thorac Surg 2003;76:1036–40.

[73] van Moorsel C, Peters G, Pinedo H. Gemcitabine: future prospects of single-agent and combination studies. Oncologist 1997;2:127–34.

[74] Patel S, Papadopoulos N, Plager C, et al. Phase II study of paclitaxel in patients with previously treated osteosarcoma and its variants. Cancer 1996;78:741–4.

[75] Maier-Lenz H, Hauns B, Haering B, et al. Phase I study of paclitaxel administered as a 1-hour infusion: toxicity and pharmacokinetics. Semin Oncol 1997; 24:S1916–9.

[76] Kelly H, Goldberg R. Systemic therapy for metastatic colorectal cancer: current options, current evidence. J Clin Oncol 2005;23:4553–60.

[77] Port J, Ng B, Ellis J, et al. Isolated lung perfusion with FUDR in the rat : pharmacokinetics and survival. Ann Thorac Surg 1996;62:848–52.

[78] Smyth N, Blades B. Selective chemotherapy of the lung during unilateral pulmonary artery occlusion with a balloon-tipped catheter. J Thorac Cardiovasc Surg 1960;40:653–66.

[79] Karakousis CP, Park HC, Sharma SD, et al. Regional chemotherapy via the pulmonary artery for pulmonary metastases. J Surg Oncol 1981;18:249–55.

[80] Wang HY, Ng B, Ahrens C, et al. Unilateral pulmonary artery occlusion inhibits growth of metastatic sarcoma in the rat lung. J Surg Oncol 1994;57:183–6.

[81] Furrer M, Lardinois D, Thormann W, et al. Cyto-static lung perfusion by use of an endovascular blood flow occlusion technique. Ann Thorac Surg 1998;65: 1523–8.

[82] Lee R, Boasquevisque C, Boglione M, et al. Isolated lung liposome-mediated gene transfer produces organ-specific transgenic expresssion. Ann Thorac Surg 1998;66:903–7.

ELSEVIER
SAUNDERS

Thorac Surg Clin 16 (2006) 199–202

THORACIC
SURGERY
CLINICS

Index

Note: Page numbers of article titles are in **boldface** type.

1547-4127/06/$ – see front matter © 2006 Elsevier Inc. All rights reserved.
doi:10.1016/S1547-4127(06)00036-3

thoracic.theclinics.com

Changing Your Address?

Make sure your subscription changes too! When you notify us of your new address, you can help make our job easier by including an exact copy of your Clinics label number with your old address (see illustration below.) This number identifies you to our computer system and will speed the processing of your address change. Please be sure this label number accompanies your old address and your corrected address—you can send an old Clinics label with your number on it or just copy it exactly and send it to the address listed below.

We appreciate your help in our attempt to give you continuous coverage. Thank you.

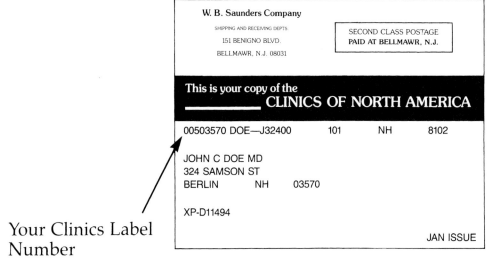

W. B. Saunders Company

SHIPPING AND RECEIVING DEPTS.

151 BENIGNO BLVD.

BELLMAWR, N.J. 08031

SECOND CLASS POSTAGE
PAID AT BELLMAWR, N.J.

This is your copy of the
CLINICS OF NORTH AMERICA

00503570 DOE—J32400   101   NH   8102

JOHN C DOE MD
324 SAMSON ST
BERLIN   NH   03570

XP-D11494

JAN ISSUE

Your Clinics Label Number

Copy it exactly or send your label
along with your address to:
W.B. Saunders Company, Customer Service
Orlando, FL 32887-4800
Call Toll Free 1-800-654-2452

Please allow four to six weeks for delivery of new subscriptions and for processing address changes.